Curing Hay Fever Naturally

with
Chinese Medicine

Bob Flaws

BLUE POPPY PRESS

Published by:
BLUE POPPY PRESS, INC.
1775 LINDEN AVE.
BOULDER, CO 80304

First Edition, November, 1997

ISBN 0-936185-91-0   LC 97-74484
COPYRIGHT 1997 © BLUE POPPY PRESS

WARNING: When following some of the self-care techniques given in this book, failure to follow the author's instruction may result in side effects or negative reactions. Therefore, please be sure to follow the author's instructions carefully for all self-care techniques and modalities. For instance, wrong or excessive application of moxibustion may cause local burns with redness, inflammation, blistering, or even possible scarring. If you have any questions about doing these techniques safely and without unwanted side effects, please see a local professional practitioner for instruction.

DISCLAIMER: The information in this book is given in good faith. However, the author and the publishers cannot be held responsible for any error or omission. The publishers will not accept liabilities for any injuries or damages caused to the reader that may result from the reader's acting upon or using the content contained in this book.

COMP Designation: Original work using a standard translational terminology

Printed at Johnson's Printing in Boulder, CO
on essentially chlorine-free paper
Cover design by Jeff Fuller of Crescent Moon

10 9 8 7 6 5 4 3 2 1

Other books in this series include:
Curing PMS Naturally with Chinese Medicine
Curing Insomnia Naturally with Chinese Medicine
Breast Health Naturally with Chinese Medicine
Curing Depression Naturally with Chinese Medicine
Curing Arthritis Naturally with Chinese Medicine

Preface

This is a layperson's book on Chinese medicine and hay fever or allergic rhinitis. The information it contains will also be very helpful for people suffering from allergic asthma. For many years, I myself suffered from allergic rhinitis, both seasonal and to animal dander, and from asthma. Since learning Chinese medicine and living by its precepts, I have not had an episode of asthma in many years and do not even own any asthma medication. I do not have hay fever, and I can even be around cats without feeling that dreaded itching in my eyes and constriction in my lungs.

Chinese medicine has helped me learn what was at the root of my allergies and how to correct especially my diet in order to eliminate my allergies' fundamental causes. As a professional practitioner of Chinese medicine, I have also helped many other Western patients overcome their allergies as well. Therefore, I know from firsthand experience what Chinese medicine has to offer sufferers of allergic rhinitis and allergic asthma, and my desire to share this valuable information with a larger audience has prompted me to write this book. If you follow the advice it contains, I believe that you too will experience fewer and less severe allergic attacks and that your general level of health and well-being will definitely improve. Good reading and good health!

Bob Flaws
Boulder, CO
May, 1997

Table of Contents

Introduction

It was spring again and Jim was not a happy camper. For several days, his nose had been running constantly, his eyes and the roof of his mouth itched incessantly, and he couldn't smell a thing. In addition, his eyes were red, he felt helpless and unattractive, and he was extremely irritable. As a child, Jim had been diagnosed as suffering from seasonal allergic rhinitis. This is the medical name for what most of us call hay fever. Its other medical name is pollinosis. Jim had to go to work today, a one hour drive in heavy traffic. Once he got to work, he was supposed to give an important presentation to the board of directors. He had tried over the counter antihistamines, but these made him feel drunk—something he could not afford this morning. What to do?

What is hay fever?

Hay fever is a group of symptoms characterized by seasonal or perennial sneezing, runny nose, nasal congestion, itching of the eyes, nose, and throat, and possible conjunctivitis or red eyes. Usually the itching starts first, followed by the runny nose, sneezing, and congestion. In Western medicine, there are three main types. Spring type is due to tree pollens, such as oak, elm, maple, alder, birch, and cottonwood. Summer type is due to grass pollens, such as bermuda, timothy, sweet vernal, orchard, and johnson grasses, and to weed pollens, such as sheep sorrel and English plantain. And fall type is due to weed pollens, such as ragweed. In some people, allergic rhinitis is due primarily to airborne fungus spores rather than to pollens. People who are allergic to these may develop the symptoms of hay fever at any time of the year. However, they are especially susceptible after damp weather, when working outside in the garden, and when working in any place where dust contains fungus, (*i.e.*, mold), spores. It is also possible to be allergic to animal dander and dust mites.

People who have hay fever also often have other types of allergic conditions, such as allergic asthma, atopic dermatitis, and hives or urticaria. For instance, some people with hay fever will go on to develop asthmatic attacks if the hay fever is either bad enough or lasts long enough. Asthma refers to difficulty breathing accompanied by wheezing and coughing. Some people also develop sinusitis or infection and inflammation of the sinus cavities secondary to a bout of hay fever. Other symptoms associated with hay fever include frontal headaches (due to sinus congestion), irritability, loss of appetite, depression, and insomnia.

Who gets hay fever?

More than 50 million Americans suffer from various types of allergies. That means one out of five! One out of every 11 office visits to a doctor is for some sort of allergy. Of this 50 million allergy sufferers, 35 million or 17% of the population have allergic rhinitis. Some authorities even place this figure as high as 20-25%. Allergic rhinitis is the single most common chronic disease experienced by Americans. Allergic rhinitis accounts for one out of 40 or 2.5% of all office visits to MDs in the United States. Fifteen million Americans or 7% of the population suffer from asthma, and the most common cause of asthma is allergies. Asthma is the number one reason for school absenteeism of all chronic diseases. It is the number six cause for hospitalization for all diseases and the number one cause for hospitalization in children. Asthma costs the U.S. economy an estimated $4.5 billion per year and as many as 5,000 Americans die from this disease each year.

Allergies affect both men and women and people of all ages. However, there is an inherited or genetic component to many

2

people's allergies. This means that one in three children will have allergies if one of their parents does, while all children will probably have allergies if both parents have allergies. In terms of asthma, children with a single asthmatic parent have a 25% likelihood of developing this disease. If both parents have asthma, the likelihood goes up to 50%. Atopy is another risk factor for asthma. Atopy is an inherited tendency to develop allergies but not a specific form. In other words, parents and children might both be allergic but not necessarily to the same things. Nearly 25% of children with asthma have more than one allergic symptom, and children who develop asthma when they're older generally have more allergic symptoms.

Aside from inheritance, it is not known in Western medicine why some people get allergies and others do not. Some believe that hormonal influences, viral infections, smoking, and a number of other influences affect whether one develops allergies. No one knows all the reasons why people with equal likelihood to develop allergies become allergic to different things, or why some have hay fever and others have asthma. What is known is that the occurrence of allergies is sharply on the rise. The number of sufferers of asthma, for instance, has jumped 61% since the early 1980s. In a recent cover story in *Newsweek* about asthma, James Wedner of the Washington University School of Medicine had this to say about the increase in allergies in developed countries:

> Why are we becoming more allergic? Ten allergists will give you 10 different answers—maybe 15 or 20. No one really knows.[1]

What causes hay fever?

People who have allergies are hypersensitive to the things that they are allergic to. When a water soluble protein molecule of the

---

[1] Wedner, James, quoted in "Why Ebony Can't Breathe", Geoffrey Cowley & Anne Underwood, *Newsweek*, May 26, 1997, p. 60

offending substance enters their system, their immune system begins a counteroffensive as if the offending molecule were a major cause of disease. The body releases various pharmacologically active substances into the system, such as histamines, leukotrienes, prostaglandins, platelet activating factor, and chemotactic factor. These substances dilate the blood vessels, increase capillary permeability, cause smooth muscle contractions, and blood and tissue eosinophilia. In people with hay fever, the offending substances, *i.e.*, airborne pollens, fungal spores, animal dander, and dust mites, affect the mucus membranes of the nasal cavity and the respiratory tract.

Allergic reactions often take place very quickly. Those who experience allergy may go outside on a bright, sunny day during the season in which they are susceptible and within 15 minutes begin having allergic symptoms. This reaction is referred to as immediate hypersensitivity. Some people also experience late-phase reactions. In this case, the site of the allergic reaction gets red, swollen, hot, and tender, causing a more prolonged reaction. The person may go out at 8 A.M. and experience a late reaction at 4 P.M. Such reactions may also last one or two days, one week, or even one month from a single allergen exposure. These kinds of late-phase reactions typically play a part in chronic asthma, rhinitis, eczema, and hives.

What about allergies to animals?

Approximately 10% of the U.S. population develops allergic rhinitis when they come in contact with certain animals. For those with asthma, the percentage jumps to 20-30%. Although many people with animal allergies think they are allergic to animal hair, it is the dander, plant and mold allergens clinging to the hair, and proteins within the animal's urine and saliva that are the problem. All animals produce dander and there is no relationship between the length of an animal's hair and its tendency to cause an allergic reaction. While many animals, including dogs, birds, and rabbits, are a primary cause of allergic reactions, the cat is the most allergenic pet, and 28% of all U.S. households have at least one cat. Approximately six million Americans are allergic to cats.

What about house dust?

House dust is a major cause of allergic rhinitis in persons with perennial or year-round symptoms. House dust is a collection of debris from many sources, including fabric fibers, human skin, human and animal dander, bacteria, cockroach parts, mold spores, food particles, and other organic and synthetic materials. While a person may be allergic to any one of these components, the major allergy-causing substance in house dust is a microscopic creature called a dust mite. Mites are members of the same family as spiders. However, dust mites are so tiny, they cannot be seen without a microscope. There are 100-500 dust mites in an average gram of house dust. These mites do not bite or otherwise transmit disease. So they pose no health risk except to people who are allergic to them. It is the protein in mites and mite feces which causes allergies in humans, and the dust mite is now thought to be the most important allergen associated with asthma.

How is allergic rhinitis diagnosed?

Usually, allergic rhinitis is diagnosed from its typical recurrent symptoms or, in other words, from the patient's history. This working hypothesis is then confirmed by physical inspection of the mucus membranes and conjunctiva in the eyes. For instance, the conjunctiva are "injected", *i.e.*, congested and red, blood-shot eyes in layperson's terms, while the mucus membranes within the nose are swollen and bluish red. The role of a particular antigen or offending substance can be determined by skin patch testing. Test solutions are made from extracts of materials that are inhaled or ingested, such as pollens, molds, house dust, etc. These test solutions are applied to scratches or shallow punctures of the skin. A positive weal-and-flare reaction is usually obvious 7-20 minutes after the extract is applied if a person is allergic to that substance.

Diagnosis is also confirmed by the presence of increased eosinophils (a type of white blood cell) in the nasal secretions and by certain antibodies in the blood, although this latter method is expensive.

How does Western medicine treat hay fever?

Antihistamines

The most common Western medical treatment of hay fever is with antihistamines. Antihistamines were developed about 50 years ago. Since the release of histamines is responsible for many of the signs and symptoms of hay fever, antihistamine or histamine blocking agents are used to suppress these symptoms. Unfortunately, one of the side effects of over the counter or non-prescription antihistamines are grogginess, drowsiness, or a feeling of being "out of it." Therefore, one should not drive, use machinery, or do any work which requires clarity and sharpness of mind. Many people find the side effects of such antihistamines very disturbing.

There is also a whole new generation of nonsedating antihistamines, such as terfenadine (Seldane ®) and astemizole (Hismanal ®). These prescription-only antihistamines do not cause such pronounced drowsiness and sedation. However, they are much more expensive than their nonprescription counterparts and they may produce life-threatening side effects when taken with certain other medications. Antihistamines, both over the counter and prescription, can aggravate glaucoma, prostatic obstruction, and certain kinds of peptic ulcers. Antihistamines also modify the effects of other drugs, such as alcohol and antidepressants.

Decongestants

Another medicine often used by sufferers of hay fever are decongestants. These medications often have just the opposite side effects of antihistamines. These tend to make people nervous and excitable when taken orally. Nasal decongestant sprays, drops, and inhalants are effective for nasal congestion, but do nothing to relieve red, itchy, irritated eyes. In any case, over the counter decongestants should not be taken for more than three days at a time, and a person's allergy season may go on for weeks.

Sympathomimetic drugs & corticosteroids

Sympathomimetic drugs taken orally can raise the blood pressure, and so these types of medication should not be used by people with hypertension. In addition, sometimes corticosteroids are used to control inflammation. However, if these are used for any length of time, they can have a number of disturbing side effects. According to Chinese medicine, corticosteroids can actually worsen one of the underlying mechanisms of allergies such as hay fever.

Allergy shots

If oral allergy medications are "poorly tolerated", (read too many side effects), or if asthma develops, then desensitization treatment or immunotherapy is often recommended. This consists of injecting an extract of the allergen under the skin in gradually increasing doses. However, the best results with this type of treatment require year round injections. A second downside of this kind of treatment is that it can provoke massive allergic reactions if the dose is not correct. In other words, it can cause very bad allergic reaction worse than what it is attempting to treat. This can include hives or urticaria all over the body, asthma, and even anaphylactic shock. In addition, immunotherapy is expensive and requires weekly office visits. Because of these drawbacks, immunotherapy is usually reserved for those with year-round or perennial allergies.

Chinese medicine as a safe & effective alternative

As seen above, the modern Western medical treatment of hay fever and other forms of allergic rhinitis is not entirely satisfactory. A UCLA Student Health Services handout on seasonal allergies says, "Most seasonal allergies are simply endured."[2] Since most people cannot avoid the offending substances, short of moving to a different environment or moving perpetually around the world to avoid spring, summer, or fall, there is room for another approach to this common but nonetheless distressing condition. Traditional Chinese medicine has a number of treatments for hay fever and other allergies which are one hundred percent free of side effects when they are prescribed and used properly.

In addition, Chinese medicine's theory about the causes and mechanisms of allergic rhinitis also are empowering in a way Western biomedicine typically is not. Knowing that one has a hair-trigger immune system which is hypersensitive to certain pollen molecules which then provoke the erroneous release of histamines and prostaglandins does not enable one to modify their diet and lifestyle in order to correct the roots of this condition on their own. The Chinese medical theory about this disease, couched as it is in every day descriptions taken from the natural world both enlighten and empower patients to make such adjustments on their own, thereby returning responsibility to the individual for their own health. So now let's turn to a brief introduction to Chinese medical theory in terms of allergic rhinitis.

---

[2] "Allergies (seasonal)", UCLA Student Health Services, http://www.saonet.ucla.edu/health/healthed/handouts/alergy.htm

Basic Chinese Medical Theory & Allergic Rhinitis

The traditional Chinese medical term for allergic rhinitis is *bi qiu*, sniveling nose. This refers to the runny nose characteristic of allergic rhinitis. In addition, nasal congestion, itchy nose, red eyes, and itchy eyes, all main symptoms of allergic rhinitis, are all also traditional Chinese disease categories. In other words, although allergic rhinitis is a modern Western medical disease category, Chinese doctors have been treating people with the symptoms which add up to allergic rhinitis for thousands of years.

The map is not the terrain

In order to understand and make sense of how Chinese medicine treats allergic rhinitis, one must first understand that Chinese medicine is a distinct and separate system of medical thought and practice from modern Western medicine. This means that one must shift models of reality when it comes to thinking about Chinese medicine. It has taken the Chinese more than 2,500 years to develop this medical system. In fact, Chinese medicine is the oldest continually practiced, literate, professional medicine in the world. As such one cannot understand Chinese medicine by trying to explain it in Western scientific or medical terms.

Most people reading this book have probably taken high school biology back when they were sophomores. Whether we recognize it or not, most of us Westerners think of what we learned about the human body in high school as "the really real" description of reality, not one possible description. However, if Chinese medicine is to make any sense to Westerners, one must be able to entertain the notion that there are potentially other valid descriptions of the human body, its functions, health, and disease. In grappling with this fundamentally important issue, it is useful to think about the concepts of a map and the terrain it describes.

If we take the United States of America as an example, we can have numerous different maps of this country's land mass. One map might show population. Another might show per capita incomes. Another might show religious or ethnic distributions. Yet another might be a road map. And still another might be a map showing political, *i.e.*, state boundaries. In fact, there could be an infinite number of potentially different maps of the United States depending on what one was trying to show and do. As long as the map is based on accurate information and has been created with self-consistent logic, then one map is not necessarily more correct than another. The issue is to use the right map for what you are trying to do. If one wants to drive from Chicago to Washington, D.C., then a road map is probably the right one *for that job* but is not necessarily a truer or "more real" description of the United States than a map showing annual rainfall.

What I am getting at here is that *the map is not the terrain*. The Western biological map of the human body is only one potentially useful medical map. It is no more true than the traditional Chinese medical map, and the "facts" of one map cannot be reduced to the criteria or standards of another *unless they share the same logic right from the beginning*. As long as the Western medical map is capable of solving a person's disease in a cost-effective, time-efficient manner without side effects or iatrogenesis (meaning doctor-caused disease), then it is a useful map. Chinese medicine needs to be judged in the same way. The Chinese medical map of health and disease is just as "real" as the Western biological map as long as when using it professional practitioners are able to solve their patients' health problems in a safe and effective way.

10

Therefore, to understand how traditional Chinese medicine treats allergic rhinitis, we first need to discuss, describe, and explain the fundamental concepts of this oldest professionally practiced, literate, holistic medical system. As a system, Chinese medicine is logical. Based on its theories, a practitioner can perform treatments that achieve the desired effect. Therefore, it is also pragmatic and scientific in its own way. However, Chinese medicine is a separate system from modern Western medicine, and, as such, cannot be explained by Western medical words or logic. In other words, to truly understand the how and why of Chinese medicine, we need to approach it on its own terms.

When first hearing the theories and concepts of Chinese medicine, the reader may find them odd and mystifying. This is only natural when we begin to look at something that not only *appears different* but *is completely different than what we have been raised to believe as true and real*. As I tell my patients, if reality is what the vast majority of people agree to be true, then the Chinese medical view of the body and what causes disease must be "true and real." Over one billion people in Asia view the body and disease according to the ideas of Chinese medicine. More importantly, the fact is that Chinese medicine has been effectively treating allergic rhinitis, asthma, and other allergies successfully and without side effects for over 2,000 years.

Yin & yang

Yin and yang are the cornerstones for understanding, diagnosing, and treating the body and mind in Chinese medicine. In a sense, all the other theories and concepts of Chinese medicine are nothing other than an elaboration of yin and yang. Most people have probably already heard of yin and yang but may have only a fuzzy idea of what these terms mean.

The concepts of yin and yang can be used to describe everything that exists in the universe, including all the parts and functions of the body. Originally, yin referred to the shady side of a hill and

11

yang to the sunny side of the hill. Since sunshine and shade are two interdependent sides of a single reality, these two aspects of the hill are seen as part of a single whole. Other examples of yin and yang are that night exists only in relation to day and cold exists only in relation to heat.. According to Chinese thought, every single thing that exists in the universe has these two aspects, a yin and a yang. Thus every thing has a front and a back, a top and a bottom, a left and a right, and a beginning and an end. However, a thing is yin or yang *only in relation to its paired complement.* Nothing is in itself yin or yang.

It is the concepts of yin and yang which make Chinese medicine a holistic medicine. This is because, based on this unitary and complementary vision of reality, no body part or body function is viewed as separate or isolated from the whole person. The table below shows a partial list of yin and yang pairs as they apply to the body. However, it is important to remember that each item listed is either yin or yang only in relation to its complementary partner. Nothing is absolutely and all by itself either yin or yang.

Yin	Yang
form	function
organs	bowels
blood	qi
inside	outside
front of body	back of body
right side	left side
lower body	upper body
cool, cold	warm, hot
stillness	activity, movement

As we can see from the above list, it is possible to describe every aspect of the body in terms of yin and yang.

Qi & blood

Qi (pronounced chee) and blood are the two most important complementary pairs of yin and yang within the human body. It is said that, in the world, yin and yang are water and fire, but, in the human body, yin and yang are blood and qi. Qi is yang in relation to blood which is yin. Qi is often translated as energy and definitely energy is a manifestation of qi. Chinese language scholars would say, however, that qi is larger than any single type of energy described by modern Western science. Paul Unschuld, perhaps the greatest living sinologist, translates the word qi as influences. This conveys the sense that qi is what is responsible for change and movement. Thus, within Chinese medicine, qi is that which motivates all movement and transformation or change.

In Chinese medicine, qi is defined as having five specific functions:

1. Defense

It is qi which is responsible for protecting the exterior of the body from invasion by external pathogens. This qi, called defensive qi, flows through the exterior portion of the body. The defensive qi plays an extremely important role in the development and prevention of allergic rhinitis. As we shall see, when this qi is weak, external pathogens can enter the body, especially in the nose and upper respiratory tract, creating the struggle between the so-called evil disease qi and the body's healthy righteous or immune qi which results in the symptoms of allergic rhinitis.

2. Transformation

Qi transforms substances so that they can be utilized by the body. An example of this function is the transformation of the food we

13

eat into nutrients to nourish the body, thus producing more qi and blood.

3. Warmth

Qi, being relatively yang, is inherently warm. One of the main functions of the qi is to warm the entire body, both inside and out. If this warming function of the qi is weak, cold may cause the flow of qi and blood to be congealed similarly to the way cold effects water to produce ice.

4. Restraint

It is qi which holds all the organs and substances in their proper place. Thus all the organs, blood, and fluids need qi to keep them from falling or leaking out of their specific pathways. If this function of qi is weak, then problems like uterine prolapse, easy bruising, urinary incontinence, or runny nose may occur.

5. Transportation

Qi provides the motivating force for all transportation in the body. Every aspect of the body that moves is moved by the qi. Hence the qi moves the blood and body fluids throughout the body. It is also qi which moves food through the stomach and the blood through its vessels.

Blood

In Chinese medicine, blood refers to the red fluid that flows through our vessels as recognized in modern Western medicine, but it also has meanings and implications which are different from those of modern Western medicine. Most basically, blood is that substance which nourishes and moistens all the body tissues. Without blood, no body tissue can function properly. In addition, when blood is insufficient or scanty, tissue becomes dry and withers.

Qi and blood are closely interrelated. It is said that, "Qi is the commander of the blood, and blood is the mother of qi." This means that it is qi which moves the blood but that it is the blood which provides the nourishment and physical foundation for the creation and existence of the qi.

In Chinese medicine, blood provides the following functions for the body:

1. Nourishment

Blood nourishes the body. Along with qi, the blood goes to every part of the body. When the blood is insufficient, function decreases and tissue atrophies or shrinks.

2. Moistening

Blood moistens the body tissues. This includes the skin, eyes, and ligaments and tendons of the body. Thus blood insufficiency can cause drying out and consequent stiffening or atrophy of various tissues throughout the body.

3. Blood provides the material foundation for the spirit or mind.

In Chinese medicine, the mind and body are not two separate things. The spirit is nothing other than a great accumulation of qi. The blood (yin) supplies the material support and nourishment for the spirit (yang) so that it accumulates, becomes bright, and stays rooted in the body. If the blood becomes insufficient, the mind can "float," causing problems like insomnia, agitation, and unrest.

Essence

Along with qi and blood, essence is one of the three most important constituents of the body. Essence is the most fundamental material the body utilizes for its growth, maturation, and reproduction. There are two forms of this essence. We inherit essence from our parents and we also produce our own essence from the food we eat, the liquids we drink, and the air we breathe.

The essence which comes from our parents is what determines our basic constitution, strength, and vitality. We each have a finite, limited amount of this inherited essence. It is important to protect and conserve this essence because all bodily functions depend upon it, and, when it is gone, we die. Thus, the depletion of essence has serious implications for our overall health and well-being. Fortunately, the essence derived from food and drink helps to bolster and support this inherited essence. This is possible if we eat healthily and do not utilize more of our qi and blood than we create each day. Then, when we sleep at night, the surplus qi and especially the blood are transformed into essence.

Fluids & humors

In addition to qi, blood, and essence, there are also various fluids and humors in the body. In actuality, fluids and humors are a yin-yang pair. Fluids are clear, thin, light, and movable, while humors are turbid, thick, heavy, and relatively immobile. In Chinese medicine, it is the qi which moves and transforms fluids. If the qi fails to move and transform fluids and humors, these may collect and turn into water dampness. Because it is qi which moves and transports liquids in the body, it is also said that liquids follow the movement of qi.

The viscera & bowels

In Chinese medicine, the internal organs have a wider area of function and influence than in Western medicine. Each organ has distinct responsibilities for maintaining the physical health and psychological well-being of the individual. When thinking about the internal organs according to Chinese medicine it is more accurate to view an organ as a network that spreads throughout the body, rather than as a distinct and separate physical organ as described by Western science. In Chinese medicine, the

16

relationship between the various organs and other parts of the body is made possible by the channel and network vessel system which we will discuss below.

Because the internal organs are conceived differently and perform different functions from their same named organs in modern Western medicine, they are referred to as the viscera and bowels. This is because, in Chinese medicine, there are five main viscera which afe relatively yin and six main bowels which are relatively yang. The five yin organs are the heart, lungs, liver, spleen, and kidneys. The six yang bowels are the stomach, small intestine, large intestine, gallbladder, urinary bladder, and a system that Chinese medicine refers to as the triple burner. All the functions of the entire body are subsumed or described under these eleven viscera and bowels. Thus Chinese medicine *as a system* does not "have" a pancreas, a pituitary gland, or the ovaries. Nonetheless, the functions of these Western organs are described within the Chinese medicine system of the five viscera and six bowels.

Visceral Correspondences

Organ	Tissue	Sense	Spirit	Emotion
Kidneys	bones/ head hair	hearing	will	fear
Liver	sinews	sight	ethereal soul	anger
Spleen	flesh	taste	thought	thinking/ worry
Lungs	skin/body hair	smell	corporeal soul	grief/ sadness
Heart	blood vessels	speech	spirit	joy/fright

The five viscera are the most important in this system. These are the organs that Chinese medicine says are responsible for the creation and transformation of qi and blood and the storage of essence. For instance, the kidneys are responsible for the excretion of urine but are also responsible for hearing, the strength of the bones including the low back, sex reproduction, maturation and growth. This points out that the Chinese organs may have the same name and even some overlapping functions but yet are quite different from the organs of modern Western medicine. Each of the five viscera also has a corresponding tissue, sense, spirit, and emotion related to it. These are outlined in the table above.

In addition, each viscus or bowel possesses both a yin and a yang aspect. The yin aspect of a viscus or bowel refers to its substantial nature or tangible form. Further, an organ's yin is responsible for the nurturing, cooling, and moistening of that viscus or bowel. The yang aspect of the viscus or bowel represents its functional activities or what it does. An organ's yang aspect is also warming. These two aspects, yin and yang, form and function, cooling and heating, create good health when they are in balance. However, if either yin or yang becomes too strong or too weak, the result will be disease.

In terms of the cause and prevention of allergic rhinitis, there are four main viscera which are important. These are the lungs, spleen, kidneys, and liver. The involvement of these four viscera in allergic rhinitis very dramatically illustrates the holistic nature of Chinese medicine. When these four viscera function properly and work together harmoniously, the body does not develop allergies. If these four viscera do not function properly, then the body is at risk to develop any of a myriad of allergies.

The lungs

Let's start with the lungs. Although the lungs are not actually the root of allergic rhinitis, most Westerners would concede that the lungs probably play a part in allergies affecting the respiratory tract. In Chinese medicine, the following statements of fact all are used to explain how allergies are caused and treated.

1. The lungs govern the qi.

In particular, the lungs govern the defensive qi. It is the defensive qi which defends the body from invasion by external pathogens.

2. The lungs are the delicate viscus.

This means that the lungs are the most susceptible to external invasion of all the viscera. It is also said that the lungs are the florid canopy. This means that the lungs are like a capstone over the other viscera and bowels. As such, they are also the first organ to be affected by externally invading pathogens floating on the wind.

3. The lungs form snivel.

Snivel is the fluid of the lungs. Therefore, lung diseases often involve some abnormality of the snivel, such as runny nose, stuffed nose, or dry nose.

4. The lungs govern the downbearing of the qi.

It is the lung qi which moves the qi of the entire body and, therefore, the body fluids propelled by the qi downward. If the lungs become diseased, qi typically counterflows upward. Upward counterflow of lung qi causes sneezing, coughing, chest oppression, and panting and wheezing or asthma. If the lung qi counterflows upward, body fluids will not descend but may rather be drafted upward along with the lung qi, resulting in runny nose. This connection between the body fluids is underscored by the saying that the lungs govern the regulation and flow through the waterways.

5. The lungs open into the portals of the nose, while the pharynx and larynx are the doors of the lungs and stomach.

This means that lung problems may cause symptoms involving the nose, pharynx, and throat. As an extension of this, when the lungs are harmonious, the nose is able to know fragrance from fetor. This means that loss of smell is a potential outcome when the lungs are diseased.

6. The lungs depend on nourishment from the spleen.

The lungs get their qi from the spleen. If the spleen is vacuous and weak, then the lung qi will also be vacuous and insufficient. However, the lungs and kidneys mutually engender each other. The lungs are the governor of the qi, while the kidneys are the root of qi. This means that the health of the lungs is also dependent on healthy kidneys. If the kidneys are weak and insufficient, so will the lung qi.

The spleen

The spleen is actually the single most important Chinese organ or viscus in terms of allergic rhinitis. The spleen and its paired bowel, the stomach, are central in the digestive process. The spleen plays a crucial role in the body's ability to transform food and drink into qi and blood. The spleen, kidneys, and lungs all play a part in the metabolism and movement of water throughout the body. However, the spleen plays the most crucial part when excessive body fluids gather and collect, transforming into dampness and thence into phlegm. Readers familiar with Western anatomy and physiology may be scratching their heads as they compare the Chinese medicine ideas of spleen function with what they know the spleen does from Western physiology. Again, they should be cautioned that Chinese medicine views the internal organs and their functions differently from Western medicine. Chinese medical statements of fact about the spleen in terms of allergic rhinitis include:

1. The spleen governs the transportation and transformation of food and water.

This means that the spleen takes the partially digested food and fluids from the stomach and begins the process of transforming it into qi, blood, and essence. A healthy spleen is vital for producing sufficient qi and blood.

2. The spleen governs the qi of the five viscera.

This saying underscores and reiterates the fact that the spleen is the source of qi for all the other viscera and bowels.

3. The spleen governs the upbearing of the clear.

The clear means the clear part of foods and liquids. Its opposite is the turbid. If the spleen functions properly, clear qi is upborne to empower the sense organs in the head and the higher mental functions. If the spleen is vacuous and weak, then the clear qi will not be upborne and the turbid qi will, consequently, not be downborne. In that case, there will not be proper production of lung and defensive qi on the one hand, while dampness and turbidity will collect and transform into phlegm on the other.

4. The spleen is averse to dampness, and the sweet flavor enters the spleen.

These two statements are important for understanding diet's impact on the spleen and its role in allergic rhinitis. Foods which are either too sweet or too damp damage the spleen and engender dampness and phlegm.

The kidneys

In Chinese medicine, the kidneys are considered the foundation of human life. Because the developing fetus looks like a large kidney and because the kidneys are the main organ for the storage of inherited essence, the kidneys are referred to as the prenatal root. Thus it is essential to good health and longevity to keep the kidney qi strong and kidney yin and yang in relative balance. The most important Chinese medical facts about the kidneys in terms of allergic rhinitis are:

1. The kidneys are responsible for human reproduction, development, and maturation.

These are the same functions we described when we discussed the essence. This is because the essence is stored in the kidneys. Health problems related to reproduction, development, and maturation are commonly problems of kidney essence. Excessive sexual activity, drug use, or simple prolonged over-exhaustion can all damage and consume kidney essence. In addition, this statement is used to explain how a disease may be inherited. It also helps explain why a person may grow out of a disease as they mature and why that disease may return as they age. In the first case, the disease goes away because of the maturation of the kidney qi, while, in the second, it returns because of the decline of the kidney qi with age.

2. The kidneys are the water viscus and the foundation of water metabolism.

They work in coordination with the lungs and spleen to insure that water is spread properly throughout the body and that excess water is excreted as urination. Therefore, problems such as edema, excessive dryness, excessive day or nighttime urination, or even runny nose can indicate a weakness of kidney function.

3. The kidneys govern opening and closing.

This means that it is the kidney qi which is responsible for the opening and closing of the body orifices. If the kidney qi becomes weak and insufficient, it may fail to hold body fluids within these portals. In that case, one may see excessive urination, excessive vaginal discharge, chronic diarrhea, or even chronic runny nose.

4. Kidney yin and yang are the foundation for the yin and yang of all the other organs and bowels and body tissues of the entire body.

This is another way of saying that the kidneys are the foundation of our life. If either kidney yin or yang is insufficient, eventually the yin or yang of the other viscera and bowels will also become insufficient.

The liver

The liver is the fourth viscus in Chinese medicine commonly involved in allergic rhinitis. This is because:

1. The liver governs the coursing and discharge of the qi.

Coursing and discharging are other words for the free flow and spreading of the qi. While the lungs (and ultimately the spleen) supply the power for the qi to move, it is the liver which allows the qi to move. Movement is an intrinsic quality of qi and movement is necessary for the qi to perform its functions. If the liver loses control over the orderly reaching or spreading of the qi, on the one hand, the qi mechanism upbearing the clear and downbearing the turbid will cease to function. On the other, qi will become depressed, stagnate, collect, and gather.

2. The liver governs upbearing effusion.

Because the qi is yang, it tends to move upward and especially if a lot of qi collects in one place. Therefore, when the liver loses its function of coursing and discharging, qi typically first backs up and accumulates and then, secondly, counterflows upward erroneously. This then may negatively affect the downbearing of the lung qi and give rise to sneezing, coughing, asthmatic panting and wheezing, headache, and red eyes, all potentially symptoms of upward counterflow of the qi. In particular, it is said that the liver opens into the portals of the eyes. This explains that eye problems often involve the liver.

3. Anger is the emotion of the liver and it damages the liver.

The liver's coursing and discharging is most easily damaged by emotional causes and, in particular, by anger, stress, and frustration. When we are frustrated, our qi wants to flow but the circumstances won't allow it. Usually, we repress our feelings in such instances and this then causes depression and constraint of the flow of qi controlled by the liver. This type of stagnation and constraint of the flow of liver qi due to emotional frustration and stress is called liver depression qi stagnation in Chinese medicine. Conversely, when the liver becomes *dis-eased*, one usually sees anger and irritability as a symptom of this.

4. The liver is yin in form but yang in function, and liver yang may transform into fire.

This saying implies that the liver has a lot of yang, remembering that qi is yang. If the qi becomes depressed and backs up in the liver, this may easily transform into heat or fire. Signs of abnormal heat in the body include sensations of heat and the color red.

5. Liver fire may invade the lungs.

This saying states that there is an especially close pathological relationship between the liver and the lungs. If depressive heat accumulates in the liver, this may counterflow into and invade the lungs. Conversely, it is also possible for lung disease and especially lung heat to stir up, engender, or aggravate liver heat.

The channels & network vessels

Each viscus and bowel has a corresponding channel with which it is connected. In Chinese medicine, the inside of the body is made up of the viscera and bowels. The outside of the body is composed of the sinews and bones, muscles and flesh, and skin and hair. It is the channels and network vessels which connect the inside and the outside of the body. It is through these channels and network vessels that the viscera and bowels connect with their corresponding body tissues.

The channels and network vessel system is a unique feature of Chinese medicine. These channels and vessels are different from the circulatory, nervous, or lymph systems. The earliest reference to these channels and vessels is in *Nei Jing (Inner Classic)*, a text written around the 2nd or 3rd century BCE.

The channels and vessels perform two basic functions. They are the pathways by which the qi and blood circulate through the body and between the organs and tissues. Additionally, the channels connect the internal organs with the exterior part of the body. This channel and vessel system functions in the body much like the world information communication network. The channels allow the various parts of our body to cooperate and interact to maintain our lives.

The channel and network vessel system is complex. There are 12 so-called regular channels, six yin and six yang, each with a specific pathway through the external body and connecting with an internal organ (see diagram). There are also extraordinary vessels, channel sinews, channel divergences, main network vessels, and ultimately countless finer and finer network vessels permeating the entire body. All of these form a closed loop or circuit that is similar to, but energetically distinct from, the circulatory system of Western medicine.

Summary

By now the reader should have appreciation for and a basic understanding of the holistic nature of Chinese medicine. In Chinese medicine, nothing stands alone. Every part and function in the body *co-responds* to other parts and functions in the body.

The body, mind, and spirit form an integrated whole. Health is the harmonious interaction of all the various aspects that comprise the organism. Disease and pain result when there is a disruption to this fundamental harmony and balance. In Chinese medicine, the focus of treatment is the restoration of harmony. Next, let's look at the Chinese medical causes and disease mechanism of allergic rhinitis.

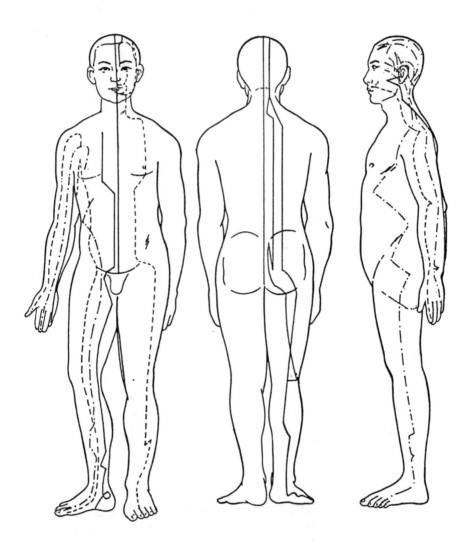

The Chinese Medical Causes of Allergic Rhinitis

All the signs and symptoms of allergic rhinitis have to do with the lungs, liver, spleen, and kidneys, with the spleen being the pivotal organ in this scenario.

Invasion by wind evils

Let's begin with the actual allergic attack or episode. In Chinese medicine, unseen disease causing agents which travel through space are referred to as wind evils. This is similar in concept to the original meaning of *malaria*, bad air. Chinese doctors in ancient times knew that there was some factor in the environment which precipitated allergic episodes. This factor cannot be seen with the naked eye, it travels through or on the air, and it attacks the upper respiratory tract. Wind evils do not mean that the person actually has been exposed to windy weather per se.

If such unseen pathogens or wind evils invade the body, they occupy the space through which the body's normal qi, blood, and body fluids flow. Since two things cannot occupy the same space, these wind evils disturb the free flow of the body's righteous healthy qi. In the case of allergic rhinitis, the specific variety of wind evils enter the body through the mouth and nose. As we have seen in the chapter above, the nose and throat are associated with the lungs. At first, the wind evils cause local congestion in the affected area. Thus one of the first symptoms of the onset of

27

allergic rhinitis is localized itching. This itching is the symptom of an impediment to the free flow of qi and blood in the affected area.

This itching is soon followed by sneezing and runny nose. As the disease evils of external "wind" enter the body more deeply they disturb the function of the first organ they come to. The lungs are the florid canopy or the capstone of all the other viscera and bowels and they are also the delicate viscus, meaning that they are relatively easily invaded by external evils. The lungs' function is to downbear the qi. If wind evils disturb the function of the lungs' clearing and downbearing, the lung qi counterflows upward, producing sneezing. Since the lungs also diffuse body fluids downward and fluids follow the movement of the qi, if the lung qi counterflows upward, fluids may spill over above from the portal associated with the lungs, the nose. Hence there is runny nose. If lung function is compromised and disturbed even more, there can be coughing and asthma.

Because of the close association of the lungs and the liver, if the lung qi counterflows upward due to disturbance by externally invading wind evils, this can also disturb the liver. If there is liver depression qi stagnation with depressive heat accumulating in the liver, this invasion by wind evils of the lungs may be all that is needed to tip the balance and allow or stimulate this depressive heat to also counterflow upward to the portal of the liver, the eyes.

The pivotal role of the spleen

Although acute allergic episodes may be triggered by invasion of the body by external wind evils, not everyone in a given environment will develop allergies. So there must be other factors besides simply the presence of external wind evils in the environment. The *Nei Jing* or *Inner Classic*, the so-called bible of Chinese medicine compiled approximately 250 BCE, says, "If evils assemble somewhere, qi must necessarily be vacuous." What this means is that evil qi cannot invade the body of a person whose defensive qi is strong and sufficient. Therefore, people with allergies are those whose defensive qi is weaker than others. Because their defensive qi is weaker than others, they are invaded by "wind evils" which do no harm to others in the same environment.

The defensive qi is manufactured out of the food and drink taken into the body through the transformation of the spleen. In other words, the root of defensive qi vacuity is mainly spleen qi vacuity. If the spleen qi is strong or fortified, the defensive qi will secure the exterior of the body from attack.

In addition, it is the spleen which mainly moves and transforms body fluids. If the spleen is vacuous and weak, it may fail in this duty. In that case, fluids may collect and transform into dampness. If this dampness endures, it will congeal into phlegm. Although the place where this phlegm is produced is in the Chinese idea of the spleen, the place where it winds up is in the lungs. Thus it is said in Chinese medicine, "The spleen is the root of phlegm engenderment, but the lungs are the place where it is stored." It is phlegm and dampness mainly due to spleen vacuity which form the mucus which runs from the nose. Therefore, in allergic rhinitis, spleen vacuity is the root of the defensive qi vacuity which allows for abnormally easy invasion and is also the root of the abnormal phlegm production.

In some people, due to inherited variability, the spleen may be constitutionally weak and vacuous. However, in Western culture, spleen vacuity is often endemic because of other factors as well. First of all, babies' spleens are inherently weak. According to Chinese medical theory, the spleen and stomach do not mature until around six years of age. If one either overfeeds infants or feeds them hard to digest foods, this further damages the spleen and engenders a lot of dampness and phlegm. This is why so many babies and young children have allergies and asthma, and often a lifetime of allergies is begun by poor feeding practices of newborns.

Overfeeding means feeding suckling infants on demand rather than on a schedule, while feeding hard to digest foods too early in life means introducing solid foods too young. In addition, some foods are either inherently damp or directly damage the spleen. Wheat and dairy products are inherently damp and, therefore, tend to engender phlegm in those with weak digestion, whereas chilled, cold, and raw foods as well as excessively sweet foods, including fruit juices, damage the spleen.

Therefore, many children develop allergies not solely due to constitutionally weak spleens but also due to damaged spleens in turn due to faulty feeding and diet. Some children will "grow out" of their allergies as their spleens mature. Other children will not, either because they are so constitutionally weak or have been damaged so badly by improper diet.

In addition, lack of sufficient exercise causes spleen vacuity and subsequent engenderment of dampness and phlegm. From the emotional point of view, Chinese medicine says that overthinking and especially worry and anxiety damage the spleen, while anger and frustration cause liver depression which then vents itself onto the spleen indirectly damaging it.

Hence there are several factors accounting for the spleen vacuity and phlegm dampness at the root of most allergic rhinitis: inherited spleen weakness, faulty diet, too little exercise, and the emotional factors of overthinking, worry, anger, and frustration. This helps explain why some peoples' allergies come and go. One spring a person's hay fever may be bad and another it may not even though the pollen counts are relatively the same. Or, for a number of years a person may be horribly allergic to cats and then "grow out of it" for several years. When they get under stress and eat badly, then their allergy may flare up again.

The kidneys' relationship with the spleen

In Chinese medicine, the spleen and kidneys are the two most important organs for proper physiological function and they mutually support and help each other. The kidneys are the former heaven or prenatal root. This means that the kidneys are the repository of the former heaven or inherited essence. The spleen is the latter heaven or postnatal root. This is because the spleen is the root of qi and blood engenderment and transformation from the food and drink we take in each day. If the spleen and stomach are like a pot on a stove distilling the finest essence of food and drink into qi and blood, then the kidneys are the ultimate source of heat under that pot. Prenatally, spleen qi is dependent on kidney yang as its root. If the spleen qi becomes weak, then eventually this will also weaken kidney yang. Conversely, if kidney yang is weak, spleen qi cannot be very strong.

In actuality, defensive qi or defensive yang is a combination of both spleen qi and kidney yang. Hence, inherited tendencies towards being allergic often involve prenatal or congenital kidney vacuity. Since the kidneys do not become exuberant and mature until after puberty, kidney vacuity also plays a part in many pediatric patients' allergies. And since the kidneys decline with age, allergies, including asthma, may worsen again after the full vigor of middle age. Because the kidney qi helps the spleen move and transform body fluids, kidney vacuity may play a part in the accumulation of phlegm dampness. In addition, the kidney qi helps the spleen qi hold the body fluids within the confines of the body. Therefore, kidney vacuity may also play a part in chronic runny nose.

The role of the liver

In the preceding chapter, we saw that it is the liver's job to keep the qi moving freely and smoothly throughout the body. If, due to emotional problems, the liver's coursing and discharging of the qi becomes inhibited, the qi will become depressed and back up.

31

Eventually, this stagnant qi has to go somewhere. According to an ancient Chinese medical teaching called five phase theory, when the liver qi becomes stagnant, it is most likely to be vented onto the spleen. When liver qi attacks the spleen, the spleen becomes vacuous and weak.

However, the liver qi may also counterflow upward assailing the lungs. Such upward counterflow of liver qi aggravates and predisposes the lung qi to also counterflow upward. Hence, if there is liver depression qi stagnation, the lungs will counterflow upward all the more easily than if there is not. This is why most patients with allergic rhinitis have a combination of spleen qi vacuity, phlegm dampness, and liver depression qi stagnation.

Because qi is yang, if it stagnates and accumulates, it tends to transform into heat. Because heat is yang, it tends to travel upwards in the body. Such a tendency for liver depression to transform into heat is aggravated by the presence of phlegm dampness which also impedes the free flow of yang qi. This depressive heat may waft up to the eyes, causing red, itchy eyes. It may also draft upward to the lungs causing what Chinese medicine calls hot or heat asthma. If it flows up to the nose and sinuses, it may cause sinusitis. If it flows up to the throat, it may cause sore, itchy throat. If this heat counterflows outward into the skin, it may cause hives with raised, red weals. Depressive heat in the liver is also experienced and manifests as easy anger or irritability.

Most people when they get sick get frustrated. Rarely does the body fail us at opportune times. Usually things go wrong just as we are about to do something either important or enjoyable. Therefore, being ill can be very frustrating. No one likes to go out in company with red, itchy eyes, a scratchy throat, a stuffed, red, runny nose with a constant need to sneeze and blow one's nose. Thus, if liver depression qi stagnation did not play a role in the creation of the allergic attack, typically it will complicate matters once the attack is under way.

32

Root & branch

In Chinese medicine, there is an important discrimination between root and branch diseases or the root and branches of a disease. Acute allergic reactions are categorized as a branch disease. When such an acute episode occurs, treatment is typically directed at relieving the branch symptoms as quickly as possible. Allergic attacks are precipitated by invasion of wind evils — unseen disease causing factors which are transmitted through the air or "on the wind."

However, the root of allergic rhinitis and allergic asthma is a combination of spleen qi vacuity with a habitual abundance of phlegm and dampness plus kidney vacuity and liver depression and also depressive possible heat. In my close to 20 years of clinical experience, this is the complicated pattern I see over and over again in sufferers of allergic rhinitis and allergic asthma. Some patients will suffer from kidney yin vacuity. Others will suffer from kidney yang vacuity. Some may not suffer from any kidney vacuity at all. Some may typically display more signs and symptoms of liver depression qi stagnation, while others may display less. In women, it is also possible to see this scenario complicated by blood vacuity, since the spleen is also the root of blood engenderment and since women lose blood every month with menstruation.

Therefore, during the remittent stage between allergic episodes, the treatment of allergic rhinitis and allergic asthma in Chinese medicine is mainly directed at supplementing the spleen and boosting the qi, transforming phlegm and eliminating dampness, supplementing kidney yin and/or yang as necessary, and coursing the liver and rectifying the qi as necessary. If there is depressive heat, then this heat is resolved and cleared in whatever organ (typically the liver and lungs and possibly the spleen and/or stomach) it is deep-lying.

33

As we will see in the chapters below, Chinese medicine has safe and effective treatments, both professionally administered and home remedies, for both acute allergic episodes and the underlying root of these episodes during the time between attacks. However, I believe that it is the teachings and techniques on treating the root of this condition which is most valuable to Western patients. When modern Western medicines are used short-term for acute episodes, they often do a satisfactory job with few serious side effects. But as we have seen above, Western medicine does not really have an answer for why certain people have certain allergies. Chinese medicine does. Based on these answers, over time, patients can change the underlying root of their condition and thus prevent the recurrence of future attacks.

I know this is possible because I had horrible hay fever and allergies to animal dander as a child, as a teenager, and as a young adult. Often episodes of allergic rhinitis would quickly progress to asthma attacks. My allergies were so bad, I had to ask potential hosts if they owned any cats. If they did, I could not enter their house. Now, however, even cats haven't been a problem for years.

How Chinese Medicine Treats Allergic Rhinitis

Treatment based on pattern discrimination, not on disease

The hallmark of professional Chinese medicine is what is known as "treatment based on pattern discrimination." Modern Western medicine bases its treatment on a disease diagnosis. This means that two patients diagnosed as suffering from the same disease will get the same treatment. Traditional Chinese medicine also takes the patient's disease diagnosis into account. However, the choice of treatment is not based on the disease so much as it is on what is called the patient's pattern, and it is treatment based on pattern discrimination which is what makes Chinese medicine the holistic, safe, and effective medicine it is.

In order to explain the difference between a disease and pattern, let us take headache for example. Everyone who is diagnosed as suffering from a headache has to, by definition, have some pain in their head. In modern Western medicine and other medical systems which primarily prescribe on the basis of a disease diagnosis, one can talk about "headache medicines." However, amongst headache sufferers, one may be a man and the other a woman. One may be old and the other young. One may be fat and the other skinny. One may have pain on the right side of her head and the other may have pain on the left. In one case, the pain may be throbbing and continuous, while the other person's pain may be very sharp but intermittent. In one case, they may also have indigestion, a tendency to loose stools, lack of warmth in their feet, red eyes, a dry mouth and desire for cold drinks, while the other person has a wet, weeping, crusty skin rash with red borders, a tendency to hay fever, ringing in their ears, and dizziness when they stand up.

In Chinese medicine just as in modern Western medicine, both these patients suffer from headache. That is their disease diagnosis. However, they also suffer from a whole host of other complaints, have very different types of headaches, and very different constitutions, ages, and sex. In Chinese medicine, the patient's pattern is made up from all these other signs and symptoms and other information. Thus, in Chinese medicine, the pattern describes *the totality of the person as a unique individual*. And in Chinese medicine, treatment is designed to rebalance that entire pattern of imbalance as well as address the major complaint or disease. Thus, there is a saying in Chinese medicine:

One disease, different treatments
Different diseases, same treatment

This means that, in Chinese medicine, two patients with the same named disease diagnosis may receive different treatments *if their Chinese medical patterns are different*, while two patients diagnosed with different named diseases may receive the same treatment *if their TCM pattern is the same*. In other words, in Chinese medicine, treatment is predicated primarily on one's pattern discrimination, not on one's named disease diagnosis. Therefore, each person is treated individually. There is no allergic rhinitis formula or allergic rhinitis herb. Nor is there any magic allergic rhinitis acupuncture point.

Treatment without side effects

Since every patient gets just the treatment which is right to restore balance to their particular body, there are also no unwanted side effects. Side effects come from forcing one part of the body to behave while causing an imbalance in some other part. The medicine may have fit part of the problem but not the entirety of the patient as an individual. This is like robbing Peter to pay Paul. Since Chinese medicine sees the entire body (and mind!) as a single, unified whole, curing imbalance in one area of the body while causing it in another is unacceptable.

In professionally practiced Chinese medicine, the two main modalities or methods of treatment are Chinese herbal medicine and acupuncture. The remainder of this chapter is devoted to Chinese herbal medicine, while the next chapter discusses acupuncture.

Chinese herbal medicine

Because different people's allergic rhinitis is due to different combinations of several Chinese disease mechanisms, professional practitioners of Chinese medicine never treat allergic rhinitis or allergic asthma with herbal "singles." In Western herbalism, singles mean the prescription of a single herb all by itself. Chinese herbal medicine is based on rebalancing patterns, and patterns in real-life patients almost always have more than a single element. Therefore, Chinese doctors almost always prescribe herbs in multi-ingredient formulas. Such formulas may have anywhere from six to eighteen or more ingredients. When a Chinese doctor reads a prescription by another Chinese doctor, they can tell you not only what the patient's pattern discrimination is but also their probable signs and symptoms. In other words, the Chinese doctor does not just combine several medicinals which are all reputed to be "good for hay fever." Rather, they carefully craft a formula whose ingredients are meant to rebalance every aspect of the patient's body-mind.

37

Getting your own individualized prescription

Since, in China, it takes not less than four years of full-time college education to learn how to do a professional Chinese pattern discrimination and then write an herbal formula based on that pattern discrimination, most laypeople cannot realistically write their own Chinese herbal prescriptions. It should also be remembered that Chinese herbs are not effective and safe because they are either Chinese or herbal. In fact, approximately 20% of the common Chinese materia medica did not originate in China, and not all Chinese herbs are completely safe. They are only safe when prescribed according to a correct pattern discrimination, in the right dose, and for the right amount of time. After all, if an herb is strong enough to heal an imbalance, it is also strong enough to create an imbalance if overdosed or misprescribed. Therefore, I strongly recommend persons who wish to experience the many benefits of Chinese herbal medicine to see a qualified professional practitioner who can do a professional pattern discrimination and write you an individualized prescription. Towards the end of this book, I will give the reader suggestions on how to find a qualified professional Chinese medical practitioner near you.

However, in order to convey a better picture of how a Chinese doctor might prescribe a complex, multi-ingredient formula for allergic rhinitis, I would like to present the following textbook description of the Chinese herbal treatment of this condition. This description is taken from *A Practical English-Chinese Library of Traditional Chinese Medicine: Clinic of Traditional Chinese Medicine (II)*.[3] The translation is my own.

---

[3] *A Practical English-Chinese Library of Traditional Chinese Medicine: Clinic of Traditional Chinese Medicine (II)*, edited by Zhang En-qin, Shanghai College of Traditional Chinese Medicine Publishing House, Shanghai, 1990, p. 986-992

Internal treatment

Main symptoms: Paroxysmal nasal itching, soreness, distention, sneezing, and a great amount of snivel which is clear and watery in consistency, intermittent nasal obstruction, greyish white, edematous nasal mucosa, and the possible accompaniment of fatigue, lack of strength, shortness of breath, disinclination to speak, reduced eating, loose stools, fear of cold and chilled limbs, lumbar soreness, many nighttime urinations, a pale red tongue with thin, white fur, and a fine pulse

Treatment principles: Fortify the spleen and boost the qi, scatter cold and open the portals or orifices

Prescription: *Bu Zhong Yi Qi Tang* (Supplement the Center & Boost the Qi Decoction) plus *Cang Er Zi San* (Xanthium Powder)

Radix Astragali Membranacei (*Huang Qi*), 18g
Radix Panacis Ginseng (*Ren Shen*), 9g
Radix Angelicae Sinensis (*Dang Gui*), 9g
Fructus Xanthii Sibirici (*Cang Er Zi*), 9g
Flos Magnoliae Liliflorae (*Xin Yi*), 9g
Herba Menthae Haplocalycis (*Bo He*), 9g
Rhizoma Cimicifugae (*Sheng Ma*), 9g
Pericarpium Citri Reticulatae (*Chen Pi*), 9g
Rhizoma Atractylodis Macrocephalae (*Bai Zhu*), 9g
mix-fried Radix Glycyrrhizae (*Gan Cao*), 9g
Radix Bupleuri (*Chai Hu*), 9g
Radix Angelicae Dahuricae (*Bai Zhi*), 15g

These are decocted in water and administered, [one pack of these ingredients at these doses per day. This formula is for treatment during an acute attack. Then, depending on the individualized patient's pattern and symptoms, this basic formula is modified with various additions and subtractions.]

39

If lung qi vacuity is marked, increase the dose of Astragalus to 30g and add Radix Ledebouriellae Divaricatae (*Fang Feng*), 9g. If there is simultaneous abdominal distention and loose stools, add Semen Dolichoris Lablab (*Bai Bian Dou*), 15g, and Semen Coicis Lachryma-jobi (*Yi Yi Ren*), 18g. If there is lumbar soreness and many nighttime urinations, add Rhizoma Curculiginis Orchioidis (*Xian Mao*), 6g, and Radix Lateralis Praeparatus Aconiti Carmichaeli (*Fu Zi*), 6g or also administer *Jin Gui Shen Qi Wan* (*Golden Cabinet* Kidney Qi Pills). If the inferior concha [of the nose] is fat and enlarged [*i.e.*, swollen], add Radix Rubrus Paeoniae Lactiflorae (*Chi Shao*), 15g, Radix Ligustici Wallichii (*Chuan Xiong*), 9g, and Fructus Liquidambaris Taiwaniae (*Lu Lu Tong*), 9g. If the amount of clear snivel is profuse, add Fructus Schisandrae Chinensis (*Wu Wei Zi*), 9g, Fructus Pruni Mume (*Wu Mei*), 9g, and Herba Asari Cum Radice (*Xi Xin*), 3g.

External treatment

1. Blow *Bi Yun San* (Jade Cloud Powder) into the nose.

Herba Centipedae (*E Bu Shi Cao*), 30g
Radix Ligustici Wallichii (*Chuan Xiong*), 30g
Flos Magnoliae Liliflorae (*Xin Yi Hua*), 6g
Herba Asari Cum Radice (*Xi Xin*), 6g
Pulvis Indigonis (*Qing Dai*), 3g

Grind these into fine powder and blow into the nose three times per day.

2. Insert *Yu Nao Shi Ruan Gao Pian* (Fish Brain Stone Soft Ointment Tablet [*i.e.*, suppository]) into the nose.

powdered Otolith Pseudosciaenae (*Yu Nao Shi*), 9g
Borneol (*Bing Pian*), 0.9g
Flos Magnoliae Liliflorae (*Xin Yi*), 6g
Herba Asari Cum Radice (*Xi Xin*), 3g

Grind into fine powder and mix with petroleum jelly. Make into soft ointment tablet and insert into the nose one time each day.

3. Massage *Ying Xiang* (LI 20) [an acupuncture point on either side of the wings of the nose] one time each day.

The above treatments are only given as examples of typical multi-ingredient Chinese herbal formulas for an acute episode of allergic rhinitis. Individual patients may receive quite different formulas depending on the main Chinese medical characteristics of their individualized pattern. However, the basic formula for internal administration (*Bu Zhong Yi Qi Tang*) is one of the most famous Chinese herbal formulas for spleen qi vacuity complicated by liver depression qi stagnation. During times of remission where one wants to treat the root of this condition, *i.e.*, spleen vacuity and liver depression, this standard formula is often a good choice.

Experimenting with Chinese patent medicines

In reality, qualified professional practitioners of Chinese medicine are not yet found in every North American community. In addition, some people may want to try to heal their allergies as much on their own as possible. More and more health food stores are stocking a variety of ready-made Chinese formulas in pill and powder form. These ready-made, over-the-counter Chinese medicines are often referred to as Chinese patent medicines. Although my best recommendation is for readers to seek Chinese herbal treatment from professional practitioners, below are some suggestions of how one might experiment with Chinese patent medicines to treat allergic rhinitis.

Cang Er Zi San

This formula is named after its main ingredient, Xanthium Seeds. It is available in North America as a desiccated, powdered extract under the name Xanthium Formula. Its ingredients include:

Fructus Xanthii Sibirici (*Cang Er Zi*)
Flos Magnoliae Liliflorae (*Xin Yi Hua*)
Radix Angelicae Dahuricae (*Bai Zhi*)
Herba Menthae Haplocalycis (*Bo He*)

All four of these ingredients dispel externally invading "wind" from the body and specifically open the nasal passageways. Therefore, this formula is for the symptomatic relief of acute allergic rhinitis. The ingredients in this formula are often added to other formulas which address the underlying root mechanisms of allergic rhinitis as in the protocol given above. Because this formula only relieves the symptoms of sneezing, nasal congestion, itchy nose, and runny nose, it is not meant to be taken between attacks. Nor will it stop these attacks from coming back again.

Bi Yan Pian

The name of this formula translates as Nose Inflammation Tablets. It is available in North America as a Chinese-made pill. Like the above formula, it is primarily for the symptomatic relief of acute allergic rhinitis. It contains the first three of the four ingredients in the formula above. However, because it also contains a number of medicinals which clear heat according to Chinese medicine, it is best when there is an element of heat in the condition. Such an element of heat would manifest as thick, opaque, white nasal mucus, yellow mucus, or even green mucus. Thus, this formula can also be used for acute sinusitis. Like the above formula, it is not a root treatment, but it can be combined with other formulas which do address the root of the problem.

Bi Min Gan Wan (also spelled Pe Min Kan Wan)

Literally, the name of these Chinese-made pills is Nasal Allergy Pills. They are for the relief of acute allergic rhinitis attacks where there is a combination of externally invading wind evils and internally engendered liver-gallbladder heat counterflowing upward. They can also be used to treat acute sinusitis. Their ingredients include:

Fructus Xanthii Sibirici (*Cang Er Zi*)
Herba Agastachis Seu Pogostemi (*Huo Xiang*)
Fel Ursi (*Xiong Dan*)
Calculus Bovis (*Niu Huang*)
Flos Chrysanthemi Indici (*Ye Ju Hua*)
Radix Angelicae Dahuricae (*Bai Zhi*)
Flos Magnoliae Liliflorae (*Xin Yi Hua*)

Qing Bi Tang (also spelled *Ching Pi Tang*)

This is yet another formula for the treatment of acute episodes of allergic rhinitis and sinusitis. Because it includes even colder, stronger ingredients for clearing heat, it is even more strongly indicated when heat is part of the patient's pattern. In this case, the heat is in the liver-gallbladder, stomach and intestines, and lungs. Besides thick yellow or green nasal mucus, there is constipation, a flushed red face, and strong thirst with a desire to drink. This formula comes as a powdered, desiccated extract. Its Chinese name means Clear the Nose Decoction. However, it is sold under the name "Pueraria Nasal Combination." Again, this formula is only for the treatment of acute episodes where there is definite inflammation. Its use should, therefore, be discontinued as soon as the attack is brought under control and symptoms of heat have mostly disappeared.

The ingredients in this formula are:

Radix Puerariae (*Ge Gen*)
Radix Ligustici Wallichii (*Chuan Xiong*)
Herba Ephedrae (*Ma Huang*)
Radix Et Rhizoma Rhei (*Da Huang*)
Ramulus Cinnamomi Cassiae (*Gui Zhi*)
Radix Albus Paeoniae Lactiflorae (*Bai Shao*)
Semen Coicis Lachryma-jobi (*Yi Yi Ren*)
Radix Platycodi Grandiflori (*Jie Geng*)
Gypsum Fibrosum (*Shi Gao*)
Flos Magnoliae Liliflorae (*Xin Yi Hua*)

Radix Glycyrrhizae (*Gan Cao*)
uncooked Rhizoma Zingiberis (*Sheng Jiang*)
Fructus Zizyphi Jujubae (*Da Zao*)

Xiao Qing Long Tang (also spelled *Hsaio Ching Lung Tang*)

The name of this formula means Minor Blue Dragon Decoction. It is available in North America as a powdered, desiccated extract under the name Minor Blue Dragon Combination. It is one of the oldest recorded formulas in Chinese medicine for the treatment of asthma. It can also be used to treat nasal obstruction, sneezing, and runny nose due to allergic rhinitis. Like the preceding formulas, it is meant for the treatment of acute allergic episodes, not for root treatment. Unlike the preceding formula, this one treats cold asthma with copious clear, white, watery phlegm. Its ingredients are:

Rhizoma Pinelliae Ternatae (*Ban Xia*)
Herba Ephedrae (*Ma Huang*)
Radix Albus Paeoniae Lactiflorae (*Bai Shao*)
Fructus Schisandrae Chinensis (*Wu Wei Zi*)
Ramulus Cinnamomi Cassiae (*Gui Zhi*)
Herba Asari Cum Radice (*Xi Xin*)
Radix Glycyrrhizae (*Gan Cao*)
uncooked Rhizoma Zingiberis (*Sheng Jiang*)

Su Zi Jiang Qi Tang (also spelled *Su Tzu Chiang Chi Tang*)

Su Zi is the name of Perilla seeds. *Jiang qi* means to downbear the qi. While *Tang* means soup or decoction. This formula is also for the treatment of allergic rhinitis and allergic asthma. However, it is more for treating the root condition rather than the branch symptoms. It treats a pattern of phlegm dampness with upward counterflow of the qi. It can be added to other root formulas described below in order to strengthen their effect of transforming phlegm, eliminating dampness, and downbearing counterflow. Available in North America as a powdered, desiccated extract, it is sold under the name Perilla Fruit Combination. Its ingredients are:

Fructus Perillae Frutescentis (*Su Zi*)
Rhizoma Pinelliae Ternatae (*Ban Xia*)
Cortex Magnoliae Officinalis (*Hou Po*)
Radix Peucedani (*Qian Hu*)
Pericarpium Citri Reticulatae (*Chen Pi*)
Radix Angelicae Sinensis (*Dang Gui*)
Ramulus Cinnamomi Cassiae (*Gui Zhi*)
Radix Glycyrrhizae (*Gan Cao*)
Fructus Zizyphi Jujubae (*Da Zao*)
uncooked Rhizoma Zingiberis (*Sheng Jiang*)

Bu Zhong Yi Qi Tang

Mentioned above under the textbook treatment of allergic rhinitis, the name of this formula translates as Supplement the Center & Boost the Qi. In this case, the center refers to the middle burner and the spleen, the most important organ in the middle burner. This is a main formula for supplementing spleen qi vacuity. However, it also includes ingredients which course the liver and rectify the qi.[4] This formula comes in the form of Chinese and American-made pills, as a tincture, and as a desiccated powdered extract.

The ingredients in this formula are:

Radix Astragali Membranacei (*Huang Qi*)
Radix Panacis Ginseng (*Ren Shen*)
Rhizoma Atractylodis Macrocephalae (*Bai Zhu*)
mix-fried Radix Glycyrrhizae (*Gan Cao*)
Radix Angelicae Sinensis (*Dang Gui*)
Radix Bupleuri (*Chai Hu*)

---

[4] When marketed as a dried, powdered extract, this formula is sold under the name Ginseng & Astragalus Combination.

Rhizoma Cimicifugae (*Sheng Ma*)
Pericarpium Citri Reticulatae (*Chen Pi*)

Xiao Yao Wan (also spelled *Hsiao Yao Wan*)

Xiao Yao Wan is one of the most common Chinese herbal formulas prescribed. Its Chinese name has been translated as Free & Easy Pills, Rambling Pills, Relaxed Wanderer Pills, and several other versions of this same idea of promoting a freer and smoother, more relaxed flow. As a patent medicine, this formula comes as pills, and there are both Chinese-made and American-made versions of this formula available over-the-counter in the North American marketplace.[5] The ingredients in this formula are:

Radix Bupleuri (*Chai Hu*)
Radix Angelicae Sinensis (*Dang Gui*)
Radix Albus Paeoniae Lactiflorae (*Bai Shao*)
Rhizoma Atractylodis Macrocephalae (*Bai Zhu*)
Sclerotium Poriae Cocos (*Fu Ling*)
mix-fried Radix Glycyrrhizae (*Gan Cao*)
Herba Menthae Haplocalycis (*Bo He*)
uncooked Rhizoma Zingiberis (*Sheng Jiang*)

This formula treats the pattern of liver depression qi stagnation complicated by blood vacuity and spleen weakness with possible dampness as well. Although this formula is not for the treatment of acute episodes of allergic rhinitis, it can be used as a root treatment between attacks. In this case, liver depression is either more important or equal in importance to spleen vacuity. If spleen vacuity is more important than liver depression, then one should use one of the other formulas below. During acute episodes of allergic rhinitis, one can combine this formula with a patent medicine which targets nasal congestion, runny nose, and sneezing more specifically.

---

[5] When marketed as a dried, powdered extract, this formula is sold under the name of Bupleurum & Tang-kuei Formula.

Dan Zhi Xiao Yao Wan

Dan Zhi Xiao Yao Wan or Moutan & Gardenia Rambling Pills is a modification of the above formula which also comes as a patent medicine in the form of pills.[6] It is meant to treat the pattern of liver depression transforming into heat with spleen vacuity and possible blood vacuity and/or dampness. The ingredients in this formula are the same as above except that two other herbs are added:

Cortex Radicis Moutan (*Dan Pi*)
Fructus Gardeniae Jasminoidis (*Shan Zhi Zi*)

These two ingredients clear heat and resolve depression.

Basically, the signs and symptoms of the pattern for which this formula is designed are the same as those for *Xiao Yao San* above plus signs and symptoms of depressive heat. These might include a reddish tongue with slightly yellow fur, a bowstring and rapid pulse, a bitter taste in the mouth, and increased irritability. This formula is also a possible choice for root treatment between attacks when there is liver depression, spleen vacuity, and definite depressive heat.

Xiao Chai Hu Tang (also spelled Hsiao Chai Hu Tang)

Sold as a powdered, desiccated extract under the name Minor Bupleurum Combination, this is probably the single most frequently prescribed Chinese herbal formula in the world. Like the above formula, it treats a combination of liver depression, spleen vacuity, and depressive heat. However, it treats depressive heat specifically in the liver, gallbladder, stomach, and lungs. It also treats an element of phlegm and not just dampness. It can be used either as a root treatment when there is liver depression,

---

[6] When marketed as a dried, powdered extract, this formula is called Bupleurum & Peony Formula.

47

spleen vacuity, heat in the liver, stomach, and lungs, and phlegm — a very common complicated pattern — or as a branch treatment if combined with one of the other patent medicines described above designed for the first aid relief of the symptoms of allergic rhinitis, such as *Bi Min Gan Wan*.

The ingredients in this formula are:

Radix Bupleuri (*Chai Hu*)
Radix Scutellariae Baicalensis (*Huang Qin*)
Radix Panacis Ginseng (*Ren Shen*)
Rhizoma Pinelliae Ternatae (*Ban Xia*)
mix-fried Radix Glycyrrhizae (*Gan Cao*)
Fructus Zizyphi Jujubae (*Da Zao*)
uncooked Rhizoma Zingiberis (*Sheng Jiang*)

Gui Pi Wan (also spelled *Kuei Pi Wan*)

Gui means to return or restore, *pi* means the spleen, and *wan* means pills. Therefore, the name of these pills means Restore the Spleen Pills.[7] However, these pills not only supplement the spleen qi but also nourish heart blood and calm the heart spirit. They are the textbook guiding formula for the pattern of heart-spleen dual vacuity. In this case, there are symptoms of spleen qi vacuity, such as fatigue, poor appetite, and cold hands and feet plus symptoms of heart blood vacuity, such as a pale tongue, heart palpitations, and insomnia. This formula is also the standard one for treating heavy or abnormal bleeding due to the spleen not containing and restraining the blood within its vessels. This patent medicine can be combined with *Xiao Yao San* when there is liver depression qi stagnation complicated by heart blood *and* spleen qi vacuity. Its ingredients are:

Radix Astragali Membranacei (*Huang Qi*)

---

[7] When sold as a dried, powdered extract, this formula is called Ginseng & Longan Combination.

Radix Codonopsitis Pilosulae (*Dang Shen*)
Rhizoma Atractylodis Macrocephalae (*Bai Zhu*)
Sclerotium Pararadicis Poriae Cocos (*Fu Shen*)
mix-fried Radix Glycyrrhizae (*Gan Cao*)
Radix Angelicae Sinensis (*Dang Gui*)
Semen Zizyphi Spinosae (*Suan Zao Ren*)
Arillus Euphoriae Longanae (*Long Yan Rou*)
Radix Polygalae Tenuifoliae (*Yuan Zhi*)
Radix Auklandiae Lappae (*Mu Xiang*)

Again, this formula is meant for root treatment between attacks.

Er Chen Wan

Er Chen Wan means Two Aged (Ingredients) Pills.[8] This is because, two of its main ingredients are aged before using. This formula is used to transform phlegm and eliminate dampness. This formula can be added to just about any formula when there is pronounced phlegm dampness. Its ingredients include:

Rhizoma Pinelliae Ternatae (*Ban Xia*)
Sclerotium Poriae Cocos (*Fu Ling*)
mix-fried Radix Glycyrrhizae (*Gan Cao*)
Pericarpium Citri Reticulatae (*Chen Pi*)
uncooked Rhizoma Zingiberis (*Sheng Jiang*)

Cautions & caveats

The above Chinese patent medicines only give a suggestion of how one or several over-the-counter Chinese ready-made preparations may be used to treat both the acute stage and root condition underlying allergic rhinitis and allergic asthma. As a professional practitioner of Chinese medicine, I prefer to see patients receive a professional diagnosis and an individually tailored prescription.

---

[8] When sold as a dried, powdered extract, this formula is called Citrus & Pinellia Combination.

However, as long as one is careful to try to match up their pattern with the right formula and not to exceed the recommended dosages, one can try treating their allergic rhinitis with one or more of these remedies. If it works, great! These patent medicines are usually quite cheap. If this approach doesn't work after one week or there are *any side effects*, one should stop and see a professional practitioner.

Six guideposts for assessing any over the counter medication

In general, you can tell if any medication and treatment are good for you by checking the following six guideposts:

1. Digestion   4. Mood
2. Elimination   5. Appetite
3. Energy level   6. Sleep

If a medication, be it modern Western or traditional Chinese, gets rid of your symptoms and all six of these basic areas of human health improve, then that medicine or treatment is probably OK. However, even if a treatment or medication takes away your major complaint, if it causes deterioration in any one of these six basic parameters, then that treatment or medication is probably not OK and is certainly not OK for long term use. When medicines and treatments, even so-called natural, herbal medications, are prescribed based on a person's pattern of disharmony, then there is healing without side effects. According to Chinese medicine, this is the only kind of true healing.

Acupuncture & Moxibustion

When the average Westerner thinks of Chinese medicine, they probably first think of acupuncture. Certainly acupuncture is the best known of the various methods of treatment which go to make up Chinese medicine. However, in China, acupuncture is actually a secondary treatment modality, most Chinese immediately thinking of "herbal" medicine when thinking of Chinese medicine.

Be that as it may, most professional practitioners of Chinese medicine in North America are licensed or otherwise registered and permitted to practice medicine as acupuncturists. Therefore, most such practitioners treat every patient with at least some acupuncture no matter if they also prescribe a Chinese herbal formula as well. While this "doubling up" of these two therapies is not always necessary to successfully treat most disease, acute allergic rhinitis and acute allergic asthma typically do respond quickly to correctly prescribed and administered acupuncture. For treating the root condition underlying allergic reactions, usually acupuncture alone is not as time or cost effective as Chinese herbal medicine alone.

What is acupuncture?

Acupuncture primarily means the insertion of extremely thin, sterilized, stainless steel needles into specific points on the body where Chinese doctors have known for centuries there are special concentrations of qi and blood. Therefore, these points are like switches or circuit breakers for regulating and balancing the flow of qi and blood over the channel and network system we described above. As we have seen, allergic rhinitis during an acute flare-up involves a localized congestion of qi and blood and upward counterflow of the lung and often the liver qi. Since acupuncture's forte is the regulation and rectification of the flow of qi, it is an especially good treatment mode for treating allergic symptoms due to qi congestion and counterflow. In that case, insertion of acupuncture needles at various points in the body moves stagnant qi and leads the qi to flow in its proper directions and amounts.

As a generic term, acupuncture also includes several other methods of stimulating acupuncture points, thus regulating the flow of qi in the body. The main other modality is moxibustion. This means the warming of acupuncture points mainly by burning dried, aged Oriental mugwort on, near, or over acupuncture points. The purpose of this warming treatment are to 1) even more strongly stimulate the flow of qi and blood, 2) add warmth to areas of the body which are too cold, and 3) add yang qi to the body to supplement a yang qi deficiency. Other acupuncture modalities are to apply suction cups over points, to massage the points, to prick the points to allow a drop or two of blood to exit, to apply Chinese medicinals to the points, to apply magnets to the points, and to stimulate the points by either electricity or laser.

What is a typical acupuncture treatment for allergic rhinitis like?

In China, acupuncture treatments are given every day or every other day, three to five times per week depending on the nature and severity of the condition. In general, it is best if one can get acupuncture every day for the first couple of treatments during one's allergy "season." Once the symptoms back off, one can begin to space out the treatments to every other day and thence to once or twice a week. After three to four weeks, the treatments should be tapered off completely.

When the person comes for their appointment, the practitioner will ask them what their main symptoms are, will typically look at their tongue and its fur, and will feel the pulses at the radial arteries on both wrists. Then, they will ask the patient to lie down on a treatment table. Based on their Chinese pattern discrimination, the practitioner will select anywhere from one to eight or nine points to be needled.

The needles used today are ethylene oxide gas sterilized, disposable needles. This means that they are used one time and then thrown away, just like a hypodermic syringe in a doctor's office. However, unlike relatively fat hypodermic needles, acupuncture needles are hardly thicker than a strand of hair. The skin over the point is disinfected with alcohol and the needle is quickly and deftly inserted somewhere typically between one quarter and a half inch. In some few cases, a needle may be inserted deeper than that, but most needles are only inserted relatively shallowly.

After the needle has passed through the skin, the acupuncturist will usually manipulate the needle in various ways until he or she feels that the qi has "arrived." This refers to a subtle but very real feeling of resistance around the needle. When the qi arrives, the patient will usually feel a mild, dull soreness around the needle, a slight electrical feeling, a heavy feeling, or a numb or tingly feeling. All these mean that the needle has "obtained" or tapped the qi and that treatment will be effective. Once the qi has been obtained, then the practitioner may further adjust the qi flow by manipulating the needle in certain ways, may attach the needle to an electroacupuncture machine in order to stimulate the point with very mild and gentle electricity, or they may simply leave the needle in place. Usually the needles are left in place from 10-20 minutes. After this, the needles are withdrawn and thrown away. *Thus there is absolutely no chance for infection from another patient.*

How are the points selected?

The points one's acupuncturist chooses to needle each treatment are selected on the basis of Chinese medical theory and the known clinical effects of certain points. Since there are different schools or styles of acupuncture, point selection tends to vary from practitioner to practitioner. However, let me present a fairly typical case from the point of view of the dominant style of acupuncture in the People's Republic of China.

Let's say the patient's main complaints are itchy eyes, itchy throat, sneezing, runny nose, nasal congestion, fatigue, irritability, chest constriction or stuffiness, and slight wheezing. Their tongue is very fat and pale with thin, white fur. Their tongue is so fat that one can clearly see the indentations of the teeth on the edges of the tongue. Their pulse is fine and bowstring. This person's Chinese pattern discrimination is wind cold invasion disturbing the lungs with upward counterflow, spleen qi vacuity, and phlegm dampness. This is a very commonly encountered Chinese pattern of disharmony in young and middle-aged adults during an acute episode of allergic rhinitis.

The treatment principles necessary for remedying this case are to resolve the exterior and dispel wind, fortify the spleen and boost the qi, rectify the qi and downbear counterflow, transform phlegm and open the portals. In order to accomplish these aims, the practitioner might select the following points:

Ying Xiang (LI 20)
Zan Zhu (Bl 2)
Lie Que (Lu 7)
He Gu (LI 4)
Tai Chong (Liver 3)
San Yin Jiao (Spleen 6)

Zu San Li (Stomach 36)
Shan Zhong (Conception Vessel 17)
Feng Men (Bl 11)
Fei Shu (Bl 12)

In this case, *Ying Xiang*, which is next to the wings of the nose opens the portal of the nose, relieves congestion, and stops sneezing and runny nose. *Zan Zhu*, at the inside corners of both eyebrows, relieves the itching of the eyes. *Lie Que* on the lung channel and *He Gu* on the large intestine channel resolve the exterior and dispel wind from the respiratory tract. The combination of *Feng Men* and *Fei Shu*, points on the upper back affecting the lungs, reinforce this action. *Shan Zhong*, on the midline of the chest between the nipples, also helps to regulate and downbear the lung qi at the same time as relieving the symptoms of stuffy chest. *Tai Chong,* a point on the liver channel, courses the liver and resolves depression, moves and rectifies the qi. It is especially effective when combined, as in this case, with *He Gu*. Together, these two points are very good for calming irritability. *San Yin Jiao*, a point on the inside of the lower legs, is chosen to further course the liver at the same time it fortifies the spleen. It does both these things because both the liver and spleen channels cross at this points. Further, this point is known to promote the nourishment and supplementation of yin blood. *Zu San Li* is the most powerful point on the stomach channel. Because the stomach is yang and the spleen is yin and because the stomach and spleen share a mutually "exterior/interior" relationship, stimulating *Zu San Li* can bolster the spleen with yang qi from the stomach which usually has plenty to spare. In addition, the stomach channel traverses the chest and, therefore, needling this point can regulate the qi in the chest.

Therefore, this combination of 10 points addresses this person's Chinese pattern discrimination and their major complaints of runny nose, stuffy nose, sneezing, itchy eyes, irritability, fatigue, and chest oppression. It remedies both the underlying disease mechanism and addresses certain key symptoms in a very direct and immediate way. Hence it provides symptomatic relief *at the same time as* it begins to correct the underlying mechanisms of these symptoms.

Does acupuncture hurt?

In Chinese, it is said that acupuncture is *bu tong*, painless. However, most patients will feel soreness, heaviness, electrical tingling, or distention. When done well and sensitively, it should not be sharp, biting, burning, or really painful.

How quickly will I feel the result?

One of the best things about the acupuncture treatment of allergic rhinitis and allergic asthma is that its effects are often immediate. Since many of the mechanisms of allergic rhinitis and asthma have to do with stuck qi, as soon as the qi is made to flow, the symptoms disappear. Therefore, many patients report they can breathe through their nose after the very first treatment.

In addition, because irritability and nervous tension are also mostly due to liver depression qi stagnation, most people will feel an immediate relief of irritability and tension while still on the table. Typically, one will feel a pronounced tranquility and relaxation within five to ten minutes of the insertion of the needles. Many patients do drop off to sleep for a few minutes while the needles are in place.

Ear acupuncture

Acupuncturists believe there is a map of the entire body in the ear and that by stimulating the corresponding points in the ear, one can remedy those areas and functions of the body. Therefore, many acupuncturists will not only needle points on the body at large but also select one or more points on the ear. In terms of allergic rhinitis and asthma, needling the points *Fei* (Lungs), *Bi* (Nose), and *Ding Chuan* (Stabilizing Asthma) can have a profound effect on relaxing bronchiole spasm and relieving nasal congestion and runny nose.

The nice thing about ear acupuncture points is that one can use tiny "press needles" which are shaped like miniature thumbtacks. These are pressed into the points, covered with adhesive tape, and left in place for five to seven days. This method can provide continuous treatment between regularly scheduled office visits. Thus ear acupuncture is a nice way of extending the duration of an acupuncture treatment. In addition, these ear points can also be stimulated with small metal pellets, radish seeds, or tiny magnets, thus getting the benefits of stimulating these points without having to insert actual needles.

The Three Free Therapies

Although one can experiment cautiously with Chinese herbal medicinals, one cannot really do acupuncture on oneself. Therefore, Chinese herbal medicine and acupuncture and its related modalities mostly require the aid of a professional practitioner. However, there are three free therapies which are crucial to treating allergic rhinitis and asthma. These are diet, exercise, and deep relaxation. Only you can take care of these three factors in your health!

Diet

We have seen that the spleen is typically the key organ in the Chinese disease mechanisms of allergic rhinitis and asthma. In Chinese medicine, the function of the spleen and stomach are likened to a pot on a stove or still. The stomach receives the foods and liquids which then "rotten and ripen" like a mash in a fermentation vat. The spleen then cooks this mash and drives off (*i.e.*, transforms and upbears) the pure part. This pure part collects in the lungs to become the qi and in the heart to become the blood. In addition, Chinese medicine characterizes this transformation as a process of yang qi transforming yin substance. All the principles of Chinese dietary therapy, including what persons with hay fever and asthma should and should not eat, are derived from these basic "facts."

We have already seen that the spleen is the root of qi and blood engenderment and transformation. Based on this fact, a healthy, strong spleen prevents and treats allergic rhinitis in three ways.

59

First, if the spleen is healthy and strong, it will create sufficient defensive qi to secure the exterior of the body from invasion by "wind evils." Secondly, since the spleen is in charge of moving and transforming water in the body, a strong, healthy spleen prevents the gathering of phlegm and dampness which then hinder the function of the lungs and easily spill over as nasal mucus. And third, the force behind the movement of the qi is mainly derived from the spleen qi which then empowers the lungs. Therefore, if the spleen qi is healthy and sufficient, there is a good push behind the movement of qi. This sufficiency of push helps counterbalance or control any tendency of the liver to constrict or constrain the qi flow. Thus, in Chinese medicine, a healthy spleen helps keep the liver in check and free from depression and stagnation.

Therefore, when it comes to Chinese dietary therapy and respiratory allergies, the two main issues are 1) to avoid foods which damage the spleen, and 2) to avoid foods which engender dampness and, therefore, phlegm.

Foods which damage the spleen

In terms of foods which damage the spleen, Chinese medicine begins with uncooked, chilled foods. If the process of digestion is likened to cooking, then cooking is nothing other than predigestion outside of the body. In Chinese medicine, it is a given that the overwhelming majority of all food should be cooked, *i.e.*, predigested. Although cooking may destroy some vital nutrients (in Chinese, qi), cooking does render the remaining nutrients much more easily assimilable. Therefore, even though some nutrients have been lost, the net absorption of nutrients is greater with cooked foods than raw. Further, eating raw foods makes the spleen work harder and thus wears the spleen out more quickly. If one's spleen is very robust, eating uncooked, raw foods may not be so damaging, but we have already seen that allergic patient's spleens are already weak. It is also a fact of life that the spleen is constitutionally weak as a youngster and inevitably weakens again with age.

60

More importantly, chilled foods directly damage the spleen. Chilled, frozen foods and drinks neutralize the spleen's yang qi. The process of digestion is the process of turning all foods and drinks to 100° Fahrenheit soup within the stomach so that it may undergo distillation. If the spleen expends too much yang qi just warming the food up, then it will become damaged and weak. Therefore, all foods and liquids should be eaten and drunk at room temperature at the least and better at body temperature. The more signs and symptoms of spleen vacuity a person presents, such as fatigue, chronically loose stools, undigested food in the stools, cold hands and feet, dizziness on standing up, and aversion to cold, the more closely they should avoid uncooked, chilled foods and drinks.

In addition, sugars and sweets directly damage the spleen. This is because sweet is the flavor which inherently "gathers" in the spleen. It is also an inherently dampening flavor according to Chinese medicine. This means that the body engenders or secretes fluids which gather and collect, transforming into dampness, in response to foods with an excessively sweet flavor. In Chinese medicine, it is said that the spleen is averse to dampness. Dampness is yin and controls or checks yang qi. The spleen's function is based on the transformative and transporting functions of yang qi. Therefore, anything which is excessively dampening can damage the spleen. The sweeter a food is, the more dampening and, therefore, more damaging it is to the spleen.

Foods which engender dampness & phlegm

Other foods which are dampening and, therefore, damaging to the spleen is what Chinese doctors call "sodden wheat foods." This means flour products such as bread and noodles. Wheat (as opposed to rice) is damp by nature. When wheat is steamed, yeasted, and/or refined, it becomes even more dampening. In addition, all oils and fats are damp by nature and, hence, may damage the spleen. The more oily or greasy a food is, the worse it

61

is for the spleen. Because milk contains a lot of fat, dairy products are another spleen-damaging, dampness-engendering food. This includes milk, butter, and cheese.

If we put this all together, then ice cream is just about the worst thing a person with a weak, damp spleen could eat. Ice cream is chilled, it is intensely sweet, and it is filled with fat. Therefore, it is a triple whammy when it comes to damaging the spleen. Likewise, pasta smothered in tomato sauce and cheese is a recipe for disaster. Pasta made from wheat flour is dampening, tomatoes are dampening, and cheese is dampening. In addition, what many people don't know is that a glass of fruit juice contains as much sugar as a candy bar, and, therefore, is also very damaging to the spleen and damp-engendering.

Below is a list of specific Western foods which are either uncooked, chilled, too sweet, or too dampening and thus damaging to the spleen. Persons with respiratory allergies should minimize or avoid these proportional to how weak and damp their spleen is.

Ice cream
Sugar
Candy, especially chocolate
Milk
Butter
Cheese
Yogurt
Raw salads
Fruit juices

Juicy, sweet fruits, such as oranges, peaches, strawberries, and tomatoes
Fatty meats
Fried foods
Refined flour products
Yeasted bread
Nuts
Alcohol (which is essentially sugar)

If the spleen is weak and wet, one should also not eat too much at any one time. A weak spleen can be overwhelmed by a large meal, especially if any of the food is hard-to-digest. This then results in food stagnation which only impedes the free flow of qi all the more and further damages the spleen.

A clear, bland diet

In Chinese medicine, the best diet for the spleen and, therefore, by extension for most humans, is what is called a "clear, bland diet." This is a diet high in complex carbohydrates such as unrefined grains, especially rice, and beans. It is a diet which is high in *lightly cooked* vegetables. It is a diet which is low in fatty meats, oily, greasy, fried foods, and very sweet foods. However, it is not a completely vegetarian diet. Most Americans, in my experience, should eat one to two ounces of various types of meat two to four times per week. This animal flesh may be the highly popular but over-touted chicken and fish, but should also include some lean beef, pork, and lamb. Some fresh or cooked fruits may be eaten, but fruit juices should be avoided. In addition, most Americans should make an effort to include more tofu and tempeh in their diets. These are two soy foods now commonly available in North American grocery stores.

If the spleen is weak, then one should eat several smaller meals rather than one or two large meals. In addition, because rice is 1) neutral in temperature, 2) it fortifies the spleen and supplements the qi, and 3) it eliminates dampness, rice should be the main or staple grain in the diet.

A few problem foods

Coffee

There are a few "problem" foods which deserve special mention. The first of these is coffee. Many people crave coffee for two reasons. First, coffee moves stuck qi. Therefore, if a person suffers from liver depression qi stagnation, temporarily coffee will make them feel like their qi is flowing. Secondly, coffee transforms essence into qi and makes that qi temporarily available to the body. Therefore, people who suffer from spleen and/or kidney vacuity fatigue will get a temporary lift from coffee. They will feel like they have energy. However, once this energy is used up, they are left with a negative deficit. The coffee has transformed some of the essence stored in the kidneys into qi. This qi has been used, and now there is less stored essence. Since the blood and essence share a common source, coffee drinking may ultimately worsen allergies associated with blood or kidney vacuities. Tea has a similar effect as coffee in that it transforms yin essence into yang qi and liberates that upward and outward through the body. However, the caffeine in black tea is usually only half as strong as in coffee.

Chocolate

Another problem food is chocolate. Chocolate is a combination of oil, sugar, and cocoa. We have seen that both oil and sugar are dampening and damaging to the spleen. Temporarily, the sugar will boost the spleen qi, but ultimately it will result in "sugar blues" or a hypoglycemic let down. Cocoa stirs the life gate fire. The life gate fire is another name for kidney yang or kidney fire, and kidney fire is the source of sexual energy and desire. It is said that chocolate is the food of love, and from the Chinese medical point of view, that is true. Since chocolate stimulates kidney fire at the same time as it temporarily boosts the spleen, it does give one rush of yang qi. In addition, this rush of yang qi does move depression and stagnation, at least short-term. So it makes sense that some people with liver depression, spleen vacuity, and kidney yang debility might crave chocolate.

Alcohol

Alcohol is both damp and hot according to Chinese medical theory. It strongly moves the qi and blood. Therefore, persons with liver depression qi stagnation will feel temporarily better from drinking alcohol. However, the sugar in alcohol damages the spleen and engenders dampness which "gums up the works," while the heat (yang) in alcohol can waste the blood (yin) and aggravate or inflame depressive liver heat.

Hot, peppery foods

Spicy, peppery, "hot" foods also move the qi, thereby giving some temporary relief to liver depression qi stagnation. However, like alcohol, the heat in spicy hot foods wastes the blood and can inflame yang. People who run cold and damp can and should eat some hot, peppery foods. However, people with signs of heat congestion, such as thick, yellow mucous, whether from the lungs or sinuses, should steer clear of hot, peppery foods.

Sour foods

In Chinese medicine, the sour flavor is inherently astringing and constricting. Therefore, people with liver depression qi stagnation should be careful not to use vinegar and other intensely sour foods. Such sour flavored foods will only aggravate the qi stagnation by astringing and restricting the qi and blood all the more. This is also why sweet and sour foods, such as orange juice and tomatoes are particularly bad for people with liver depression and spleen vacuity. The sour flavor astringes and constricts the qi, while the sweet flavor damages the spleen and engenders dampness.

Diet sodas

In my experience, diet sodas seem to contain something that damages the Chinese idea of the kidneys. They may not damage the spleen the same way that sugared sodas do, but that does not mean they are healthy and safe. I say that diet sodas damage the kidneys since a number of my patients over the years have reported that, when they drink numerous diet sodas, they experience terminal dribbling, urinary incontinence, and low back and knee soreness and weakness. When they stop drinking diet sodas, these symptoms disappear. Taken as a group, in Chinese medicine, these are kidney vacuity symptoms. Since many sufferers of respiratory allergies and especially chronic asthma tend to suffer from concomitant kidney vacuity (along with liver depression and spleen vacuity), I typically recommend such patients to steer clear of diet sodas so as not to weaken their kidneys any further or faster.

Some last words on diet

In conclusion, Western patients are always asking me what they should eat in order to cure their disease. However, when it comes to diet, sad to say, the issue is not so much what to eat as what not to eat. Diet most definitely plays a major role in the cause and perpetuation of many people's respiratory allergies, but, except in the case of vegetarians suffering from blood or yin vacuities, the issue is mainly what to avoid or minimize, not what to eat. Most of us know that coffee, chocolate, sugars and sweets, oils and fats, and alcohol are not good for us. Most of us know that we should be eating more complex carbohydrates and freshly cooked vegetables and less fatty meats. However, it's one thing to know these things and another to follow what we know.

To be perfectly honest, a clear bland diet *à la* Chinese medicine is not the most exciting diet in the world. It is the traditional diet of most lower and lower middle class peoples around the world living in temperate climates. It is the traditional diet of most of my readers' great grandparents. The point I am making here is that our modern Western diet which is high in oils and fats, high in sugars and sweets, high in animal proteins, and proportionally high in uncooked, chilled foods and drinks is a relatively recent aberration, and you can't fool Mother Nature. I believe that one of the single greatest causes of the rise in allergic diseases is the overly rich diet of rich, industrialized nations.

When one switches to the clear, bland diet of Chinese medicine, at first one may suffer from cravings for more "flavorful" food. These cravings are, in many cases, actually associated with food allergies. In other words, we may crave what is actually not good for us similar to a drunk's craving alcohol. After a few days, these cravings tend to disappear and we may be amazed that we don't miss some of our convenience or "comfort" foods as much as we thought we would. If one has been addicted to a food like sugar for many years, it does not take much to "fall off the wagon" and be addicted again. Therefore, perseverance is the key to longterm success. As the Chinese say, a million is made up of nothing but lots of ones, and a bucket is quickly filled by steady drips and drops.

Exercise

Exercise is the second of what I call the three free therapies. According to Chinese medicine, regular and adequate exercise has three basic benefits for sufferers of respiratory allergies. First, exercise promotes the movement of the qi and quickening of the blood. Since most respiratory allergies involve qi counterflow caused or at least aggravated by qi stagnation, it is obvious that exercise is an important therapy for coursing the liver and rectifying the qi.

Secondly, exercise benefits the spleen. The spleen's movement and transportation of the digestate is dependent upon the "qi mechanism." The qi mechanism describes the function of the qi in upbearing the pure and downbearing the turbid parts of digestion. For the qi mechanism to function properly, the qi must be flowing normally and freely. Since exercise moves and rectifies the qi, it also helps regulate and rectify the qi mechanism. This then results in the spleen's movement and transportation of foods and liquids and its subsequent engendering and transforming of the qi and blood.

If the spleen qi is fortified and sufficient, then the defensive qi will be strong and secure the body from external invasion by wind evils. In addition, a strong, healthy spleen is capable of moving and transforming water in the body. Allergic rhinitis and asthma both involve phlegm and fluids collecting in, impeding the function of, and potentially overflowing from the lungs. Thus insuring that the spleen is strong and healthy insures that dampness will not collect and congeal into phlegm.

Therefore, adequate exercise is a vitally important component of any person's regime for treating the root causes of allergic rhinitis and asthma.

What kind of exercise is best for allergic rhinitis?

Aerobics

In my experience, I find aerobic exercise to be the most beneficial for most people with respiratory allergies. By aerobic exercise, I mean any physical activity which raises one's heartbeat 80% above their normal resting rate and keeps it there for at least 20 minutes. To calculate your normal resting heart rate, place your fingers over the pulsing artery on the front side of your neck. Count the beats for 15 seconds and then multiply by four. This gives you your beats per minute or BPM. Now multiply your BPM by .8. Take the resulting number and add it to your resting BPM. This gives you your aerobic threshold of BPM. Next engage in any physical activity you like. After you have been exercising for five minutes, take your pulse for 15 seconds once again at the artery on the front side of your throat. Again multiply the resulting count by four and this tells you your current BPM. If this number is less than your aerobic threshold BPM, then you know you need to exercise harder or faster. Once you get your heart rate up to your aerobic threshold, then you need to keep exercising at the same level of intensity for at least 20 minutes. In order to insure that one is keeping their heart beat high enough for long enough, one should recount their pulse every five minutes or so.

Depending on one's age and physical condition, different people will have to exercise harder to reach their aerobic threshold than others. For some, simply walking briskly will raise their heart beat 80% above their resting rate. For others, they will need to do calisthenics, running, swimming, raquetball, or some other, more strenuous exercise. It really does not matter what the exercise is as long as it raises your heart beat 80% above your resting rate and keeps it there for 20 minutes. However, there are two other criteria that should be met. One, the exercise should be something that is not too boring. If it is too boring, then you may have a hard time keeping up your schedule. Since most people do find aerobic exercises such as running, stationary bicycles, and stair-steppers boring, it is good to listen to music or watch TV in order to distract your mind from the tedium. Secondly, the type of exercise should not cause any damage to any parts of the body. For instance, running on pavement may cause knee problems for some people. Therefore, you should pick a type of exercise you enjoy but also one which will not cause any problems.

When doing aerobic exercise, it is best to exercise either every day or every other day. If one does do their aerobics at least once every 72 hours, then its cumulative effects will not be as great. Therefore, I recommend my patients with hay fever and allergies to do some sort of aerobic exercises every day or every other day, three to four times per week *at least*. The good news is that there is no real need to exercise more than 30 minutes at any one time. Forty-five minutes per session is not going to be all that much better than 25 minutes per session. And 25 minutes four times per week is very much better than one hour once a week.

Exercise induced asthma

Although exercise does not bring on episodes of allergic rhinitis, exercise can induce asthma attacks in some people. Therefore, if one has asthma, one should be careful about embarking in any new exercise regime. My advice to such people is to exercise at first at a lesser intensity that what will provoke an attack. In the meantime, really clean up one's diet. Avoid foods which damage the spleen and foods which engender dampness and phlegm. As one's signs and symptoms associated with spleen and kidney vacuity or with phlegm dampness begin to disappear, gradually introduce more strenuous exercise. Typically, one will be surprised to find that exercise becomes less and less likely to trigger an asthma attack.

Deep relaxation

As we have seen above, allergic rhinitis and asthma are commonly associated with liver depression qi stagnation. Even though this may not be the pivotal disease mechanism, it is usually a major contributory mechanism. If liver depression endures or is severe, it typically transforms into heat or fire. Heat or fire, being yang, tend to waft upward, collecting in the canopy above, the lungs. This heat may be hidden most of the time, but becomes apparent when some other factor pushes it over the edge. In Chinese medicine, heat from a depressed liver not only tends to collect in the lungs, it is also commonly transmitted to the stomach and gallbladder. The stomach and gallbladder channels both traverse the head over the location of the sinuses. Therefore, sinusitis usually involves heat in the liver and lungs as well as the stomach and gallbladder channels.

In Chinese medicine, liver depression comes from not fulfilling all one's desires. But no adult in the real world can fulfill all their desires. This is why a certain amount of liver depression is endemic among adults. When our desires are frustrated, our qi becomes depressed. This then creates emotional depression and easy anger or irritability. In Chinese medicine, anger is nothing other than the venting of pent up qi in the liver. When qi becomes depressed in the liver, it accumulates like hot air in a balloon. Eventually, that hot, depressed, angry qi has to go somewhere. So when there is a little more frustration or stress, then this angry qi in the liver vents itself as irritability, anger, shouting, or nasty words, and it moves upward in the body. In Chinese medicine, it is a basic statement of fact that, "Anger results in the qi ascending."

Essentially, this type of anger and irritability are due to a maladaptive coping response that is typically learned at a young age. When we feel frustrated or stressed, stymied by or angry about something, most of us tense our muscles and especially the muscles in our upper back and shoulders, neck, and jaws. At the same time, many of us will hold our breath. In Chinese medicine, the sinews are governed by the liver. This tensing of the muscles, *i.e.*, the sinews, constricts the flow of qi in the channels and network vessels. Since it is the liver which is responsible for the coursing and discharging of this qi, such tensing of the sinews leads to liver depression qi stagnation. Because the lungs govern the downward spreading and movement of the qi, holding our breath due to stress or frustration only worsens this tendency of the qi not to move and, therefore, to become depressed in the Chinese medical idea of the liver.

Therefore, deep relaxation is the third of the three free therapies. For deep relaxation to be therapeutic medically, it needs to be more than just mental equilibrium. It needs to be somatic or bodily relaxation as well as mental repose. Most of us no longer recognize that every thought we think and feeling we feel is actually a felt physical sensation somewhere in our body. The words we use to describe emotions are all abstract nouns, such as anger, depression, sadness, and melancholy. However, in Chinese medicine, *every emotion is associated with a change in the direction or flow of qi.* As we have said above, anger makes the qi move upward. Fear, on the other hand, makes the qi move downward. Therefore, anger "makes our gorge rise" or "blows our top", while fear may cause a "sinking feeling" or make us "pee in our pants." These colloquial expressions are all based on the age-old wisdom that all thoughts and emotions are not just mental but also bodily events. This is why it is not just enough to clear one's mind. Clearing one's mind is good, but for really marked therapeutic results, it is even better if one clears one's mind at the same time as relaxing every muscle in the body as well as the breath.

Guided deep relaxation tapes

The single most efficient and effective way I have found for myself and my patients to practice such mental and physical deep relaxation is to do a daily, guided, progressive, deep relaxation audiotape. What I mean by guided is that a narrator on the tape leads one through the process of deep relaxation. Such tapes are progressive since they lead one through the body in a progressive manner, first relaxing one body part and then moving on to another. For instance, the narrator may say something to the effect that, as you exhale, you should feel your forehead get heavy and relaxed, softening and expanding, becoming warm and heavy. As you exhale again, now feel your cheeks get heavy and relaxed, softening and expanding, becoming warm and heavy. Breathe in and breathe out, letting your breath go without hindrance or hesitation. Breathing out, now feel your jaw muscles become heavy and relaxed, expanding and softening, becoming warm and heavy, etc., etc., throughout the entire body until one comes to the bottoms of one's feet.

There are innumerable such tapes on the market. These are usually sold in health food stores, New Age music and supply stores, or in bookstores with a good selection of New Age books. Over the years of suggesting this method of deep relaxation to my patients, I have found that each patient will have his or her own preferences in terms of the type of voice, male or female, the choice of words and imagery, whether there is background music or not, and the actual pace of the progression through the body, some narrators speaking a slightly different rate and rhythm. Therefore, I suggest listening to and even purchasing more than one such tape. One should find a tape which they like and can listen to without internal criticism or comment, going along like a cloud in the sky as the narrator's voice blows away all your mental and bodily stress and tension. If one has more than one tape, one can also switch every now and again from tape to tape so as not to become bored with the process or desensitized to the instructions.

72

Key things to look for in a good relaxation tape

In order to get the full therapeutic effect of such deep relaxation tapes, there are several key things to check for. First, be sure that the tape is a guided tape and not a subliminal relaxation tape. Subliminal tapes usually have music and any instructions to relax are given so quietly that they are not consciously heard. Although such tapes can help you feel relaxed when you do them, ultimately they do not teach you how to relax as a skill which can be consciously practiced and refined. Secondly, make sure the tape starts from the top of the body and works downward. Remember, anger makes the qi go upward in the body, and people with irritability and easy anger due to liver depression qi stagnation already have too much qi rising upward in their bodies. Such depressed qi typically needs not only to be moved but also downborne. Third, make sure the tape instructs you to relax your physical body. If you do not relax all your muscles or sinews, the qi cannot flow freely and the liver cannot be coursed. Depression is not resolved, and there will not be the same medically therapeutic effect. And lastly, be sure the tape instructs you to let your breath go with each exhalation. One of the symptoms of liver depression is a stuffy feeling in the chest which we then unconsciously try to relieve by sighing. Letting each exhalation go completely helps the lungs push the qi downward. This allows the lungs to control the liver at the same time as it downbears upwardly counterflowing angry liver qi.

The importance of daily practice

When I was an intern in Shanghai in the People's Republic of China, I was once taken on a field trip to a hospital clinic where they were using deep relaxation as a therapy with patients with high blood pressure, heart disease, stroke, migraines, and insomnia. The doctors at this clinic showed us various graphs plotting their research data on how such daily, progressive deep relaxation can regulate the blood pressure and body temperature and improve the appetite, digestion, elimination, sleep, energy,

73

and mood. One of the things they said has stuck with me for 15 years: "Small results in 100 days, big results in 1,000." This means that if one does such daily, progressive deep relaxation *every single day for 100 days*, one will definitely experience certain results. What are these "small" results? These small results are improvements in all the parameters listed above: blood pressure, body temperature, appetite, digestion, elimination, sleep, energy, and mood. If these are "small" results, then what are the "big" results experienced in 1,000 days of practice? The big results are a change in how one reacts to stress—in other words, a change in one's very personality or character.

What these doctors in Shanghai stressed and what I have also experienced both personally and with my patients is that it is vitally important to do such daily, guided, progressive deep relaxation every single day, day in and day out for a solid three months at least and for a continuous three years at best. If one does such progressive, somatic deep relaxation every day, one will see every parameter or measurement of health and well-being improve. If one does this kind of deep relaxation only sporadically, missing a day here and there, it will feel good when you do it, but it will not have the marked, cumulative therapeutic effects it can. Therefore, perseverance is the real key to getting the benefits of deep relaxation.

The real test

Doing such a daily deep relaxation regime is like hitting tennis balls against a wall or hitting a bucket of balls at a driving range. It is only practice; it is not the real game itself. Doing a daily deep relaxation regime is not only in order to relieve one's immediate stress and strain. It is to learn a new skill, a new way to react to stress. The ultimate goal is to learn how to breathe out and immediately relax all one's muscles in the body in reaction to stress, rather than the common but unhealthy maladaption to stress of holding one's breath and tensing one's muscles. By doing such deep relaxation day after day, one learns how to relax any

74

and every muscle in the body quickly and efficiently. Then, as soon as one recognizes they are feeling frustrated, stressed out, or uptight, they can immediately remedy those feelings at the same time as coursing their liver and rectifying their qi. This is the real test, the game of life. "Small results in 100 days, big results in 1,000."

Finding the time

If you're like me and most of my patients, you are probably asking yourself right now, "All this is well and good, but when am I supposed to find the time to eat well-balanced cooked meals, exercise at least every other day, and do a deep relaxation every day? I'm already stretched to the breaking point." I know. That's the problem.

As a clinician, I often wish I could wave a magic wand over my patients' heads and make them all healthy and well. I cannot. After close to two decades of working with thousands of patients, I know of no easy way to health. There is good living and there is easy living. Or perhaps I am stating this all wrong. What most people take as the easy way these days is to continue pushing their limits continually to the max. The so-called path of least resistance is actually the path of lots and lots of resistance. Unless you take time for yourself and find the time to eat well, exercise, and relax, no treatment is going to eliminate your allergies completely. There is simply no pill you can pop or food you can eat that will get rid of the root causes of allergic diseases: poor diet, too little exercise, and too much stress.

Even Chinese herbal medicine and acupuncture can only get their full effect if the diet and lifestyle is first adjusted. Sun Si-maio, the most famous Chinese doctor of the Tang dynasty (618-907 CE), who himself refused government office and lived to be 101, said: "First adjust the diet and lifestyle and only secondarily give herbs and acupuncture." Likewise, it is said today in China, "Three parts treatment, seven parts nursing." This means that any cure is only 30% due to medical treatment and 70% is due to nursing, meaning proper diet and lifestyle.

In my experience, this is absolutely true. Seventy percent of all disease will improve after three months of proper diet, exercise, relaxation, and lifestyle modification. Seventy percent! Each of us has certain nondiscretionary rituals we perform each day. For instance, you may always and without exception find the time to brush your teeth. Perhaps it is always finding the time to shower. For others, it may be always finding the time each day to eat lunch. And for 99.999% of us, we find time, no, we make the time to get dressed each day. The same applies to good eating, exercise, and deep relaxation. Where there's a will there's a way. If your allergies are bad enough, you can find the time to eat well, get proper exercise, and do a daily deep relaxation tape.

The solution to allergies is in your hands

In Boulder, CO where I live, we have a walking mall in the center of town. On summer evenings, my wife and I often walk down this mall. Having treated so many patients over the years, it is not unusual for me to meet former patients on these strolls. Frequently when we say hello, these patients begin by telling me they are sorry they haven't been in to see me in such a long time. They usually say this apologetically as if they have done something wrong. I then usually ask if they've been alright. Often they tell me: "When my such-and-such flares up, I remember what you told me about my diet, exercise, and lifestyle. I then go back to doing my exercise or deep relaxation or I change my diet, and then my symptoms go away. That's why I haven't been in. I'm sorry."

However, such patients have no need to be sorry. This kind of story is music to my ears. When I hear that these patients are now able to control their own conditions by following the dietary and lifestyle advice I gave them, I know that, as a Chinese doctor, I have done my job correctly. In Chinese medicine, the inferior doctor treats disease after it has appeared. The superior doctor prevents disease before it has arisen. If I can teach my patients how to cure their symptoms themselves by making changes in their diet and lifestyle, then I'm approaching the goal of the high class Chinese doctor — the prevention of disease through patient education.

The professional practice of medicine is a strange business. We doctors are always or at least should be engaged in putting ourselves out of business. Therefore, patients have no need to apologize to me when they tell me they now have control over their health and disease in their own hands.

To get these benefits, one must make the necessary changes in eating and behavior. In addition, allergies and asthma are not a condition that is cured once and forever like measles or mumps. When I say Chinese medicine can cure allergic rhinitis and asthma, I do not mean that you will never experience a runny nose or chest oppression again. What I mean is that Chinese medicine can eliminate or greatly reduce your symptoms *as long as you keep your diet and lifestyle together*. People being people, we all "fall off the wagon" from time to time and we all "choose our own poisons." I do not expect perfection from either my patients or myself. Therefore, I am not looking for a lifetime cure. Rather, I try to give my patients an understanding of what causes their disease and what they can do to minimize or eliminate its causes and mechanisms. It is then up to the patient to decide what is bearable and what is unbearable or what is an acceptable level of health. The Chinese doctor will have done their job when *you know how to correct your health to the level you find acceptable given the price you have to pay*.

Simple Home Remedies for Hay Fever

Although faulty diet, lack of adequate exercise, and too much stress are the ultimate causes of most allergies according to Chinese medicine and, therefore, diet, exercise, and deep relaxation are the most important parts of every person's treatment and prevention of allergic rhinitis and asthma, there are a number of simple Chinese home remedies to help relieve the symptoms of respiratory allergies and improve one's general level of health.

Moxibustion

As mentioned in chapter 5, moxibustion is the burning of a Chinese herb, Folium Artemisiae Argyii (*Ai Ye*) or Mugwort, on, near, over, or under an acupuncture point or body part. While acupuncture needles act like circuit breakers and shunt the qi around the grid of the body, they cannot add any qi to the system. Moxibustion can not only warm the body but actually add yang qi to the body. Before a person can have allergies, their defensive qi must be relatively weak. It is a defensive qi vacuity which allows wind evils to penetrate the body and disturb the function of the lungs. Therefore, self-treatment with moxibustion can be used to supplement the defensive qi of the body and thus help prevent invasion by wind evils.

There are several methods of doing moxibustion. However, the safest, easiest, and most effective for adding yang qi to the body at home is to use what are called *Ibiki* moxas. These are small, ready-made cones of moxa on self-adhesive platforms manufactured in Japan. These ready made cones contain the right amount of Mugwort and the platforms prevent any potential for burning oneself. The adhesive backing prevents the moxa from falling off in the middle of the procedure.

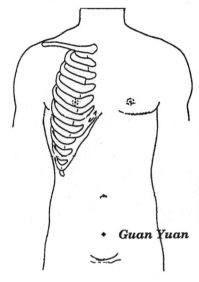

Guan Yuan

If one wants to supplement the yang qi of the body, one of the best ways to do this is to moxa two of the most powerful points in the body: *Guan Yuan* (CV 4) and *Zu San Li* (St 36). *Guan Yuan* is a point on the conception vessel. It is located four finger widths below the navel on the centerline of the lower abdomen. This point connects directly to the kidneys which are the root of all yang in the body. Moxaing this point invigorates kidney yang which then supports and fortifies the spleen qi.

Begin by locating this point while lying down on your back in a comfortable position. Stick an *Ibiki* moxa on the point and light it with a match or lit incense stick. As the moxa cone burns down, if you feel any burning heat, lift the cone off the skin. You want to turn the skin flushed red and warm under the moxa cone, but you do not want to raise a blister. Only burn one cone the first day. The second day, burn two cones. Each day, as long as you have not burned yourself, add another cone until you get up to five. Then do this every day for a month *before* the season you normally experience allergies in. If your allergies are perennial, you may do this at any time of the year, although Chinese medical theory says the juncture between summer and fall is the best time for this therapy. That occurs according to the Chinese medical calendar beginning in the first week of August.

After moxaing *Guan Yuan* from
one to five cones, next moxa
Zu San Li. This is one of the most
powerful acupoints on the body.
Moxaing this point strongly
supplements the spleen and
stomach qi. This point is located
three finger widths below the
bottom édge of the kneecap
on the outside of the lower legs
between the tibia and fibula.

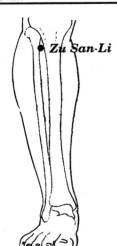

Place an *Ibiki* moxa on one *Zu San Li*
and burn it the same as on *Guan Yuan*.
You want a strong heat, but it should not be burning or blistering
hot. The first day, only burn one cone. The second day, if all went
well, burn two cones. Each day after that, burn three *Ibiki* cones
on *Zu San Li* on each leg.

Always be sure to do this technique in this order—*Guan Yuan*
first and *Zu San Li* second. By combining these two points, you
will be supplementing the kidneys and the spleen, the two viscera
involved in the production of the defensive qi. If you think you
have burned yourself, apply *Ching Hong Wan* burn ointment
available from China Herb Co. whose address is given below. If
you raise a blister, cover this with a sterile dressing and keep
clean to avoid infection. Actually, in premodern China, it was
thought that raising a blister gets one an even better result. In
that case, one does not keep moxaing every day. Instead one lets
the blister heal before moxaing again.

Ibiki moxa cones can be purchased from:

Oriental Medical Supply (OMS) Co.
1950 Washington St.
Braintree, MA 02184
Tel: (617) 331-3370 or 800-323-1839 Fax: (617) 335-5779

This method is for treating the underlying root of most allergies—a spleen-kidney vacuity. It is not for first aid treatment of allergic rhinitis or asthma during an attack. If the above directions on how to do this are not sufficiently clear for you to feel confident doing this, then you can go to a local acupuncturist who can teach you how to locate these points and do this technique at home.

Cupping

Cupping is an ancient method of healing dating back to neolithic times when animal horns were used instead of glass and porcelain cups. Basically, this technique consists of creating a vacuum on the skin. Because of this vacuum, qi and blood are pulled to an acupuncture point or area of the body.

In order to do this at home, find an empty glass jar the size of a baby food jar. Hold a small piece of cotton in a pair of needle-nosed pliers or forceps. Dip the cotton in a little rubbing alcohol. Do not get the cotton so wet that it is completely sodden and drips. Lie on your back with your navel exposed. Bring the mouth of the jar down close next to the skin surrounding your navel. Light the alcohol impregnated cotton ball and quickly swish it around the inside of the jar. It will burn out the oxygen and create a vacuum. Just before the flame of the lit cotton goes out, pull the cotton ball out of the jar and affix the mouth of the jar over the navel. If you have coordinated this correctly, the jar will be stuck to your abdomen with a firm seal. Your navel and the surrounding skin will have been sucked up into the mouth of the jar and the skin should be turning red.

Leave the jar on for three-five minutes and then remove by pressing down on one side of the jar. As soon as air creeps under the edge, the seal will be broken. Do this again three times in succession for a total of 15 minutes. Repeat this every day for 10 days.

This method is a very effective home remedy for treating all kinds of allergies, including allergic rhinitis, asthma, and hives. It can be done either before in order to prevent or during the allergy season in order to eliminate allergic reactions. Again, if these written directions do not seem enough to feel confident doing this technique, see a local acupuncturist who can quickly and easily teach you how to do it. It may turn your navel red or even lightly black and blue for a few days, but it really is an effective way for treating allergic conditions. The acupuncture point located in the center of the navel is connected to both the spleen and the kidneys and supplements both of these at the same time. Cups made in China specifically for this therapy can also be purchased from Oriental Medical Supply (OMS) Co.

Chinese self-massage

Massage, including self-massage, is a highly developed part of traditional Chinese medicine. In most traditional Chinese hospitals, there are massage wards where patients can receive treatment for almost every disease. The following Chinese self-massage regime can be used to treat acute cases of allergic rhinitis with runny nose, nasal congestion, and sore, red, itchy eyes.

1. Opening heaven's gate:
Push upward along the
midline of the forehead
from the midpoint between
the eyebrows to the anterior
hairline with the index and
middle fingers of both hands.
Begin at the level of the
eyebrows and alternately push
upward to the hairline again and
again, 50-100 times, pushing
in one direction only, from the
eyebrows upward to the hairline.

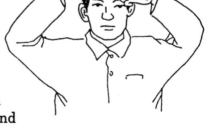

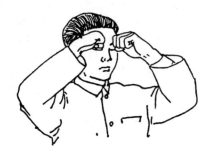

2. Pushing apart the forehead: Bend the two index fingers and push with the lateral sides of their middle segments from the midline of the forehead to the anterior hairline on both sides of the forehead and the ends of the eyebrows. Do this approximately 100 times.

3. Kneading *Tai Yang* (M-HN-9): Press with the tip of the thumbs or middle fingers on the points *Tai Yang* located in the center of each temple. Knead them approximately 100 times until there is a sensation of mild soreness and distention.

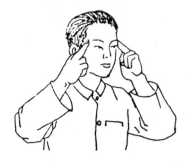

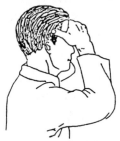

4. Wiping the temples: Press the temples with the pads of the thumbs and wipe backwards repeatedly with force approximately 100 times until there is a sensation of mild soreness and distention.

5. Pressing and kneading *Feng Chi* (GB 20): With the tips of both thumbs, press and knead the paired points *Feng Chi,* located in the depression between the upper portion of the sternocleidomastoid muscles and the trapezius, approximately one inch into the hairline, 100 times. The force should be strong enough to make the forehead sweat.

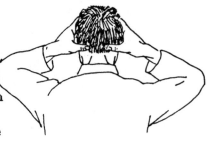

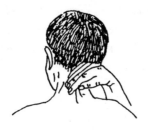

6. Grasping the muscles on both sides of the nape of the neck: Put the thumb of one hand on one side of the nape of the neck and the index and middle fingers on the other, grasping the muscles of both sides from the posterior hairline to the base of the neck 10-20 times.

7. Grasping and pounding *Jian Jing* (GB 21): With the thumb, index, and middle fingers of the left hand, grasp the right *Jian Jing*, located at the midpoint of the top of the shoulder muscle, 3-5 times. Then switch hands and grasp the left *Jian Jing* with the right hand. Next, pound the point with an empty fist 30-50 times on each side.

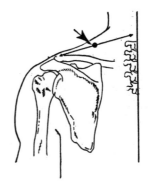

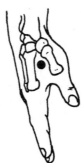

8. Patting the back: With a hollow palm, pat the opposite side of the upper back 30-50 times on each side.

9. Nipping and kneading *He Gu* (LI 4): With the nail of the opposite thumb, nip and knead the point *He Gu*, located at the midpoint of the mound of muscle between the thumb and index finger on the back of the hand, approximately 100 times each side.

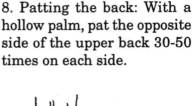

85

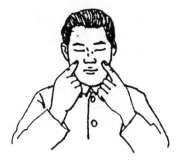

10. Knead *Ying Xiang* (LI 20): Knead the points on either side of the wings of the nose with the tips of the middle fingers approximately 100 times.

This treatment is for use during an acute allergic attack. Even just the last two maneuvers can be helpful in relieving the symptoms of an acute allergic episode.

In order to supplement the spleen and kidneys, the underlying root of most respiratory allergies, the following regime can be done daily between allergic attacks.

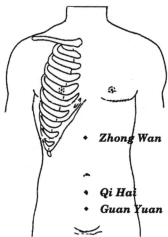

Zhong Wan

Qi Hai

Guan Yuan

1. Pressing and kneading *Zhong Wan* (CV 12), *Qi Hai* (CV 6), and *Guan Yuan* (CV 4): With one palm, press and knead the midpoint of the upper abdomen, the point 1.5 inches below the navel, and the midpoint of the lower abdomen approximately 100 times each.

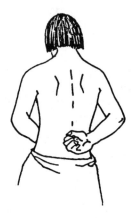

2. Pounding the lumbar region: With hollow fists, pound the entire low back region, the mansion of the kidneys, 30-50 times.

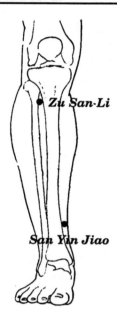

3. Pressing and kneading *Zu San Li* (St 36): With the tips of both thumbs, press and knead *Zu San Li*, located three inches below the lower outside corner of the kneecap, approximately 100 times each.

4. Pressing and kneading *San Yin Jiao* (Sp 6): With the tips of both thumbs, press and knead the points located three inches above the tip of the inner ankles just behind the tibia 50-100 times each side.

The key to getting a good effect from Chinese self-massage in terms of building up one's bodily constitution is persevering daily practice. Even just rubbing the abdomen after meals can improve the spleen and stomach function. For more Chinese self-massage regimes, the reader should see Fan Ya-li's *Chinese Self-massage Therapy: The Easy Way to Health* also published by Blue Poppy Press.

Seven star hammering

A seven star hammer is a small hammer or mallet with seven small needles embedded in its head. Nowadays in China, it is often called a skin or dermal needle. It is one of the ways a person can stimulate various acupuncture points without actually inserting a needle into the body. Seven star hammers can be used either for people who are afraid of regular acupuncture, for children, or for those who wish to treat their condition at home.

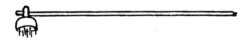

When the points to be stimulated are on the front of the body, this technique can be done by oneself. When they are located on the back of the body, this technique can be done by a family member or friend. This is a very easy technique which does not require any special training or expertise.

During an acute attack of allergic rhinitis or asthma, begin by tapping the nape of the neck, with the most tapping between the second to fourth cervical vertebrae. Also tap the region of *Feng Chi* (GB 20). This point is located behind the ears just below the base of the skull in the depression between the strap muscles of the spine and the attachment of the sternocleidomastoid muscles at the mastoid process.

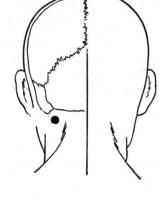

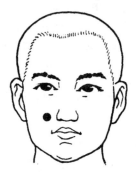

Then tap *Ying Xiang* (LI 20) on both sides of the wings of the nose.

Follow this by tapping *He Gu* (LI 4). This point is located in the center of the mound between the thumb and index fingers on the back of the hand.

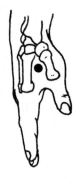

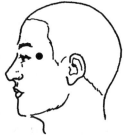

If there are red, itchy, painful eyes or headache, tap *Tai Yang* (M-HN-9). This point is located right in the center of the temple.

If there is asthma, add the entire upper back region between the spine and inside edges of the shoulder blades, the front and back intercostal spaces, both sides of the trachea or windpipe, the lower edge of the xiphoid process just below the center of the ribs, and *Tai Yuan* (Lu 9). This point is located just distal to the styloid process at the insides of the wrists. Use moderate to heavy tapping.

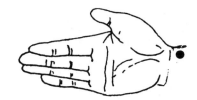

If there is any bleeding, wipe the area with a cotton swab moistened in alcohol. Then take a dry cotton ball and press the area.

To strengthen the system between allergic attacks, one can tap more lightly the following areas once per day or once every other day:

1. Both sides of the entire spinal column from the sacrum to the base of the skull

2. *Zhong Wan* (CV 12):
The center of the upper abdomen

3. *Qi Hai* (CV 6): One and a half inches below the navel on the midline of the lower abdomen

4. *Guan Yuan* (CV 4):
The center of the lower abdomen

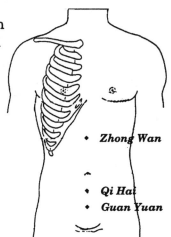

89

5. *Zu San Li* (St 36): Three inches below the lower, outer corner of the kneecap. See the picture on p. 87 for the location of this point.

Between treatments, soak the seven star hammer in alcohol or hydrogen peroxide and do not share hammers between people in order to prevent any infection from one person to another. Seven star hammers are very cheap. So each person can easily afford to have their own. They can also be purchased from OMS whose address and phone numbers are given in the section on moxibustion above.

Chinese medicinal porridges

If all food and liquids taken into the stomach must be turned into soup before the rest of digestion can take place, then eating soups and porridges is a very nutritious way of getting the most out of one's food. In other words, eating soups and porridges is predigestion, and this helps a vacuous, weak spleen. Therefore, in Chinese medicine, there are numerous medicinal recipes combining a few simple herbs with rice and making medicinal porridges. These can be used to treat acute attacks of allergic rhinitis and asthma and to build up the system and treat the root in between attacks. In English, such Chinese medicinal porridges are often referred to as congees.

Jie Cai Zhou (Mustard Greens Congee)

fresh Mustard greens, *i.e.*, Herba Sinapis Junceae (*Jie Cai*), 60g
Polished Rice, *i.e.* , Semen Oryzae Sativae (*Jing Mi*), 100g

First wash and cut the mustard greens. Then cook these and the rice in water to make into a dilute rice soup. Eat warm two times per day. This formula is for the treatment of cold phlegm cough and asthma, in which case the phlegm is clear and watery, as in most cases of simple allergic rhinitis. It diffuses the lungs and sweeps away phlegm, warms the center and boosts the stomach, resolves the exterior and disinhibits urination.

Su Ye Xing Ren Zhou (Perilla Leaf & Apricot Seed Congee)

Folium Perillae Frutescentis (*Zi Su Ye*), 9g
Semen Pruni Armeniacae (*Xing Ren*), 9g
Pericarpium Citri Reticulatae (*Chen Pi*), 6g
Polished Rice, *i.e.*, Semen Oryzae Sativae (*Jing Mi*), 50g

Boil the first three ingredients in water, remove the dregs, and add the remaining liquid to the rice. Cook the rice into porridge with this liquid and eat. This formula is for wind cold rhinitis, bronchitis, and asthma. It resolves the exterior and transforms phlegm, downbears counterflow and stops coughing and sneezing. If one does not have all four ingredients, one can still make a medicinal congee with only the last three or even just the Semen Pruni and rice.

Hu Tao Zhou (Walnut Congee)

Walnuts, *i.e.*, Semen Juglandis Regiae (*Hu Tao Ren*), 50g
Polished Rice, *i.e.*, Semen Oryzae Sativae (*Jing Mi*), 50g

Pound the walnuts into a mash and add water to the rice and cook into porridge. After the porridge is cooked, add the walnut mash and mix thoroughly. Skim off any oil on the top of the porridge and eat the remaining congee warm one time each morning and evening. This formula supplements the kidneys, boosts the lungs, and stabilizes panting, *i.e.*, asthma, and coughing. It can be used to treat the root of lung, spleen, kidney allergic rhinitis and asthma. It is not for first aid use during an acute attack.

Chong Cao Zhou (Cordyceps Congee)

Cordyceps Sinensis (*Dong Chong Xia Cao*), 6g
Polished Rice, *i.e.*, Semen Oryzae Sativae (*Jing Mi*), 50g

First cook the rice into porridge. Powder the Cordyceps and add to the cooked congee. Mix thoroughly and cook a short time more. Eat warm two times per day. Five to seven days equal one course of treatment. This formula boosts the lungs and supplements the kidneys, enriches yin and stops panting, *i.e.*, asthma. It can be used to bank the root in lung, spleen, kidney allergic rhinitis and asthma.

For numerous more Chinese medicinal porridge formulas for respiratory problems and asthma, see my *The Book of Jook, Chinese Medicinal Porridges: A Healthy Alternative to the Typical Western Breakfast* also published by Blue Poppy Press.

Chinese medicinal teas

When patients go to a professional practitioner of Chinese medicine, they will usually come away with an herbal formula with a dozen or more ingredients. They will usually also be instructed to boil these ingredients into a very strong decoction for 45 minutes to an hour or more. However, there is also folk Chinese herbal medicine which is closer in form to Western herbal medicine and which can be experimented with at home. Many of the ingredients used in folk Chinese herbal medicine are commonly available even in the West, and more and more health food stores are beginning to carry bulk Chinese herbs.

The following Chinese medicinal tea formulas are good examples of Chinese folk herbalism. You can try them if there is no Chinese doctor in your area. They are for the relief of the symptoms of an acute attack of allergic rhinitis.

Cang Er Zi Cha (Xanthium Tea)

Fructus Xanthii Sibirici (*Cang Er Zi*), 12g
Flos Magnoliae Liliflorae (*Xin Yi Hua*), 6g
Radix Angelicae Dahuricae (*Bai Zhi*), 6g
Herba Menthae Haplocalycis (*Bo He*), 6g

Tea leaves, *i.e.*, Folium Camelliae Theae (*Cha Ye*), 2g

Grind these five ingredients into powder and steep in boiling water for 10 minutes. Use one packet per day. Drink this warm repeatedly any time of the day. This formula resolves the exterior and dispels wind, opens the portals of the nose and eliminates dampness.

Xin Yi Cha (Magnolia Flower Tea)

Flos Magnoliae Liliflorae (*Xin Yi Hua*), 2g
Folium Perillae Frutescentis (*Zi Su Ye*), 6g

Grind the above two ingredients into a coarse powder, wrap in cheesecloth or put in a tea ball, and soak in boiling water. Drink this as a tea, one packet per day. This formula dispels wind, scatters cold, and frees the portals of the nose.

Bai Zhi Jing Jie Cha (Angelica & Schizonepeta Tea)

Radix Angelicae Dahuricae (*Bai Zhi*), 30g
Herba Seu Flos Schizonepetae Tenuifoliae (*Jing Jie Sui*), 3g
Tea leaves, *i.e.*, Folium Camelliae Theae (*Cha Ye*), 3g

Grind the first two ingredients into a fine powder. Steep the tea leaves in boiling water. Using this beverage wash down 6g of this powder two times per day. This formula dispels wind and scatters cold, resolves the exterior and stops pain. It treats wind cold external invasions with nasal congestion, clear, runny nose, and headache, where headache is a main symptom.

Ju Hua Long Jing Cha (Chrysanthemum & Dragon Well Tea)

Flos Chrysanthemi Morifolii (*Ju Hua*), 10g
Dragon Well Tea, *i.e.*, Folium Camelliae Theae (*Long Jing Cha*), 3g

Steep these two ingredients in boiling water for 5-10 minutes. Use one packet per day, drunk as a tea at any time. This formula treats red, itchy eyes due to a combination of wind and heat.

The next two Chinese folk teas are for treating the underlying root of respiratory allergies and asthma. The first is designed to help eliminate phlegm dampness. The second is in order to supplement the spleen and kidneys and thus prevent asthma due to spleen-kidney vacuity weakness.

Ju Cha (Tangerine Tea)

Tea leaves, *i.e.*, Folium Camelliae Theae (*Cha Ye*), 2g
dry Tangerine peel, *i.e.*, Pericarpium Citri Reticulatae (*Ju Pi*), 2g

Place these two ingredients in a cup, pour in boiling water, and steep for 10 minutes. Stops cough and transforms phlegm, rectifies the qi and harmonizes the stomach. Frequent drinking of this tea can help reduce or eliminate phlegm dampness.

Ren Shen Hu Tao Cha (Ginseng & Walnut Tea)

Radix Panacis Ginseng (*Ren Shen*), 4g
Walnuts, *i.e.*, Semen Juglandis Regiae (*Hu Tao Ren*), 4 pieces

Pound the Ginseng and walnuts into pieces, place them in a pot, and boil with water over a slow fire. This should make 400ml of concentrated liquid. Drink one packet per day, taken at any time. The Ginseng and walnut can also be chewed and eaten. This tea fortifies the spleen and supplements the kidneys, absorbs the qi[9] and levels panting. This formula is suitable for treating the root

---

[9] In Chinese medicine, the kidneys grasp or absorb the qi sent down by the lungs on inhalation. Asthma due to kidney vacuity is due, at least in part, to the kidneys being too weak to grasp or absorb this qi which then counterflows back upwards as panting and coughing.

of chronic asthma due to spleen-kidney vacuity. It is used between acute attacks in order to bank the root.

For more information on Chinese medicinal teas, see Zong Xiaofan and Gary Liscum's *Chinese Medicinal Teas: Simple, Proven Folk Formulas for Common Diseases & Promoting Health* also published by Blue Poppy Press. The medicinals in all the formulas in this chapter can be purchased by mail from:

China Herb Co.
165 W. Queen Lane
Philadelphia, PA 19144
Tel: 215-843-5864 Fax: 215-849-3338 Orders: 800-221-4372

When using any Chinese medicinal in any form, if there are any side effects, stop immediately and seek a consultation with a professional practitioner of Chinese medicine.

Creating a personalized regime

One does not need to do all these home treatments for every case of hay fever. Rather, one should select several of them as the severity of their disease, time, and personal inclination suggest. If one is already taking care of the "Three Free Therapies", it is easy to add moxibustion or cupping and a choice of Chinese medicinal teas and/or porridges. If one doesn't have the patience or discipline to do Chinese self-massage, but a partner is willing to do seven star hammering, then one might choose this therapy instead. In other words, it all depends on how severe one's allergies are and what materials one has at one's disposal.

Given the several different Chinese self-therapies in this chapter, no one should be unable to find the materials or the time to put at least one of these into practice. In some light cases of allergic rhinitis, that may be all it takes. While in more difficult, stubborn cases, one may have to do a couple or three of these to insure a good result.

95

Chinese Medical Research on Respiratory Allergies

Considerable research has been done in the People's Republic of China on the effects of acupuncture and Chinese herbal medicine on allergic rhinitis and asthma. Usually, this research is in the form of a clinical audit. That means that a group of patients with the same diseases, patterns, or major complaints are given the same treatment for a certain period of time. After this time, the patients are counted to see how many were cured, how many got a marked effect, how many got some effect, and how many got no effect. This kind of "outcome-based research" has, up until only very recently, not been considered credible in the West where, for the last 30 years or so, the double-blind, placebo-controlled comparison study has been considered the "gold standard." However, such double-blind, placebo-controlled comparison studies are impossible to design in Chinese medicine and do not, in any case, measure effectiveness in a real-life situation.

Clinical audits, on the other hand, do measure actual clinical satisfaction of real-life patients. Such clinical audits may not exclude the patient's trust and belief in the therapist or the therapy as an important component in the result. However, real-life is not as neat and discreet as a controlled laboratory experiment. If the majority of patients are satisfied with the results of a particular treatment and there are no adverse side effects to that treatment, then that is good enough for the Chinese

97

doctor, and, in my experience, that is also good enough for the vast majority of my patients.

Below are abbreviated translations of several recent research articles published in Chinese medical journals on the treatment of allergic rhinitis and asthma. These research articles exemplify how Chinese medicine treats one of the most common yet distressing complaints. I think that most persons reading these statistics would think that Chinese medicine was worth a try. Even better results can be expected when treatments are even more finely tuned to the individual patient as is the case in private practice here in the West.

From "The Treatment of 42 Cases of Allergic Rhinitis with *Si Wu Tang Jia Wei* (Four Materials Decoction with Added Flavors)" by Li Guang-zhen, *Ji Lin Zhong Yi Yao (Jilin Chinese Medicine & Medicinals)*, #3, 1993, p. 25

Since 1985, the author has treated 42 cases of allergic rhinitis with *Si Wu Tang Jia Wei*. Of these 42, 29 were men and 13 were women. They ranged in age from 19 to 62 years of age. The shortest course of disease was 4 months and the longest was 10 years. Runny nose, itchy nose, and sneezing were the main symptoms. Examination revealed that the nasal mucosa were either an ashen white or purplish, sooty color, the nasal concha was edematous, and the nasal cavity was producing a flowing secretion. Examination of the nasal secretions were positive for eosinophils.

Treatment method:

The medicinals consisted of: Uncooked Radix Rehmanniae (*Sheng Di*), 24g, Radix Angelicae Sinensis (*Dang Gui*), Radix Rubrus Paeoniae Lactiflorae (*Chi Shao*), 15g ea., Radix Ligustici Wallichii (*Chuan Xiong*), 6g, Fructus Xanthii (*Cang Er Zi*), Flos Magnoliae Liliflorae (*Xin Yi*), 9g ea., Herba Pycnostelmae (*Xu Chang Jing*),

30g. If there was headache, Radix Angelicae Dahuricae (*Bai Zhi*) and Flos Chrysanthemi Morifolii (*Ju Hua*) were added. If there was a common cold, these medicinals were combined with *Yu Ping Feng San* (Jade Windscreen Powder). One *ji*[10] was decocted per day with 15 days equaling one course of treatment. Two to four courses of treatment were given with a follow-up survey conducted one year after treatment.

Treatment outcomes:

Twenty-three patients were completely cured. This meant that their symptoms disappeared, their nasal mucosa and secretions returned to normal, and their nasal secretions tested negative for eosinophils. Thirteen cases got fair improvement. This meant that their symptoms were obviously reduced or partially disappeared. The number of attacks or the duration of attacks was also reduced, and their nasal secretions mostly tested negative for eosinophils. And six patients got no result from this treatment. This meant that there was no apparent change in their condition from before the treatment was begun. Therefore, the total effectiveness rate was 85.7%.

Discussion:

According to the author, the main Chinese medicine disease mechanism of this disease is yin and blood insufficiency. In that case, constructive and defensive are empty and sparse and the exterior defensive fails to secure. This then allows for external invasion of wind cold, and this results in the portals of the lungs (*i.e.*, the nose) losing their disinhibition. *Si Wu Tang* enriches yin

---

[10] A *ji* literally means a prescription. However, when used as it is in these research reports, a *ji* means a single packet of medicinals the doses of whose ingredients have been given above. Mostly, one *ji* is a one day dose. However, because this is typically given in two or more divided doses, to translate this word as dose could give an erroneous idea.

and nourishes blood, moves the qi and harmonizes the constructive, thus supporting the righteous. As the saying goes, "When the blood is harmonious (or harmonized), wind is automatically extinguished." Xanthium, Flos Magnoliae, and Pynostelma diffuse the lungs, open the portals, and, therefore, dispel evils. When evils are dispelled, the righteous is at ease. With the righteous returned and evils removed, the disease obtains a cure.

From "The Treatment of 100 Cases of Allergic Rhinitis with *Bu Zhong Yi Qi Tang Jia Wei* (Supplement the Center & Boost the Qi Decoction with Added Flavors)" by Feng Bi-qun & Lu Ji-sen, *Xin Zhong Yi (New Chinese Medicine)*, #6, 1995, p. 55

Since 1988, the authors have treated 100 patients suffering from allergic rhinitis with *Bu Zhong Yi Qi Tang Jia Wei* with good success. Of those 100 patients, 62 were males and 38 were females. The youngest was 13 and the oldest was 58 years old with most cases falling between 16-40. The disease course had lasted for less than 1 year in 17 cases, for 1-10 years in 77 cases, and for more than 10 years in 6 cases. The clinical manifestations were recurrent sneezing, runny nose, nasal congestion, and nasal itching. Examination of the nasal mucosa revealed that they were edematous, colored a somber white or an ashen grey and that there was usually a great amount of clear, watery snivel.

Treatment method:

The formula was comprised of: Radix Astragali Membranacei (*Huang Qi*), Radix Codonopsitis Pilosulae (*Dang Shen*), mix-fried Radix Glycyrrhizae (*Zhi Gan Cao*), Rhizoma Atractylodis Macrocephalae (*Bai Zhu*), Pericarpium Citri Reticulatae (*Chen Pi*), Radix Angelicae Sinensis (*Dang Gui*), Rhizoma Cimicifugae (*Sheng Ma*), Radix Bupleuri (*Chai Hu*), Fructus Xanthii Sibirici (*Cang Er Zi*), Flos Magnoliae Liliflorae (*Xin Yi Hua*)

The doses of these ingredients depended upon what was appropriate for the individual and the formula was modified following the patterns. If there was an exterior pattern, Radix Ledebouriellae Divaricatae (*Fang Feng*), fresh Bulbus Allii Fistulosi (*Cong Bai*), and Semen Praeparatus Sojae (*Dan Dou Chi*) were added. If yang vacuity was marked, Radix Lateralis Praeparatus Aconiti Carmichaeli (*Fu Zi*), Herba Epimedii (*Yin Yang Huo*), and Fructus Rosae Laevigatae (*Jin Ying Zi*) were added. If there was simultaneous yin vacuity, Herba Dendrobii (*Shi Hu*), Rhizoma Polygoni Odorati (*Yu Zhu*), and Fructus Ligustri Lucidi (*Nu Zhen Zi*) were added.

Definition of treatment outcomes:

Complete cure was defined as the disappearance of sneezing, runny nose, nasal congestion, nasal itching, and other such symptoms. There was no edema of the nasal passageways and no inflammatory secretion. After one year there was no relapse. Some effect was defined as marked decrease in the symptoms, no obvious nasal mucosal edema or inflammatory secretion, but recurrence once in a while in the next year. No effect meant that there was no obvious change from before to after treatment.

Treatment outcomes:

Based on the above criteria, there were 62 cures with another 30 patients getting some effect. Eight cases experienced no results from this protocol. Thus the total effectiveness rate was 92%.

Discussion:

According to the authors, allergic rhinitis is a commonly seen disease with a long course and is difficult to cure. In Chinese medicine, it is categorized as runny snivel disorder. Due to lung qi vacuity, the interstices are loose. Thus wind cold lodges in the nasal cavity. The lung qi loses its free flow and fluids and humors collect and gather. The nasal cavity becomes congested and blocked, and therefore there is sneezing and runny nose. However, the repletion and fullness of the lung qi is dependent on the transportation of the spleen qi. Therefore, *Bu Zhong Yi Qi Tang* is used to fortify the spleen and boost the qi, upbear the clear and transform dampness. This is based on banking earth to engender metal. Xanthium and Flos Magnoliae are added to assist in acridly scattering wind and cold, opening and disinhibiting the portal of the lungs. This then strengthens and increases the treatment effect.

From "The Treatment of 65 Cases of Allergic Rhinitis with *Jia Jian Xiao Chai Hu Tang* (Modified Minor Bupleurum Decoction)" by Kuang Nai-jia, Bi Guo-mei & Huang Ya-shan, *He Nan Zhong Yi (Henan Chinese Medicine)*, #5, 1995, p. 275-278

From January 1991 to July 1993, the authors treated 65 cases of allergic rhinitis with modified *Xiao Chai Hu Tang* with very good results. They began with a group of 130 patients and divided them in half into treatment and comparison groups. Of the 65 patients in the treatment group, 35 were men and 30 were women. They ranged in age from 18-65 years old and their disease course had lasted from 1-9 years. Ten patients had a mild degree of disease, 25 a moderate degree, and 30 patients had a severe degree of disease. In the comparison group, there were 36 men and 29 women. They ranged in age from 17-66 years old and they had been ill from 1–10 years. Nine patients in that group had a mild degree of disease, 26 a moderate degree, and 30 a severe degree of disease. Thus these two groups were very similar statistically (P⟨ 0.05).

Treatment method:

Xiao Chai Hu Tang consisted of: Radix Bupleuri (*Chai Hu*), 12g, Radix Scutellariae Baicalensis (*Huang Qin*), 9g, Radix Panacis Ginseng (*Ren Shen*), mix-fried Radix Glycyrrhizae (*Zhi Gan Cao*),

6g ea., uncooked Rhizoma Zingiberis (*Sheng Jiang*), 3 slices, Fructus Zizyphi Jujubae (*Da Zao*), 4 pieces. One *ji* was decocted in water each day and given warm in two divided doses. This was continued for four weeks.

If there was nasal itching and especially heavy sneezing, Flos Magnoliae Liliflorae (*Xin Yi Hua*) and Flos Chrysanthemi Morifolii (*Ju Hua*) were added. If there was relatively profuse runny nose with clear snivel, Rhizoma Atractylodis (*Cang Zhu*) and Rhizoma Cimicifugae (*Sheng Ma*) were added. If the nasal conchae were markedly swollen and distended, Radix Angelicae Dahuricae (*Bai Zhi*) and Herba Menthae Haplocalycis (*Bo He*) were added. If there was nasal cavity hyperemia and particularly heavy inflammatory reactions, Rhizoma Coptidis Chinensis (*Huang Lian*) and Radix Ligustici Wallichii (*Chuan Xiong*) were added. If there were polyps in the nasal conchae, Semen Pruni Persicae (*Tao Ren*) and Radix Puerariae (*Ge Gen*) were added. If there was accompanying accessory nasal sinusitis, Radix Salviae Miltiorrhizae (*Dan Shen*) and Rhizoma Coptidis Chinensis (*Huang Lian*) were added. If there was accompanying headache, Rhizoma Ligustici Wallichii (*Chuan Xiong*) and Radix Et Rhizoma Ligustici Chinensis (*Gao Ben*) were added. If there was accompanying itchy eyes and tearing and spring/summer catarrhal conjunctivitis, Radix Astragali Membranacei (*Huang Qi*), Flos Chrysanthemi Morifolii (*Ju Hua*), and Radix Ledebouriellae Divaricatae (*Fang Feng*) were added. If there was accompanying bronchial asthma, Cortex Radicis Mori Albi (*Sang Bai Pi*) and Radix Platycodi Grandiflori (*Jie Geng*) were added. If there was accompanying tinnitus, ear oppression, or deafness, Radix Angelicae Sinensis (*Dang Gui*), Rhizoma Alismatis (*Ze Xie*), and Rhizoma Acori Graminei (*Chang Pu*) were added.

The comparison group was given 4mg of chlorpheniramine three times each day. At the same time, both groups used Benadryl liquid nose drops. No other systemic medicinals were used.

103

Treatment outcomes:

Effectiveness was based on subjective changes in sneezing, runny nose, and nasal obstruction as well as on objective changes in the nasal mucosa. Of the treatment group, 34 cases experienced marked effect, 25 some effect, and 6 no effect. Thus the total effectiveness of this protocol in the treatment group was 90.8%. Fifty-nine of these patients were followed up after two years and only seven of these or 11.9% had a recurrence. In the comparison group, 29 experienced marked effect, 21 some effect, and 15 no effect for a total effectiveness rate of 76.9%. Fifty of these patients were followed up after two years and 16 cases or 32% had relapses. Thus there was a marked statistical difference between these two groups in terms of the effectiveness of protocols ($X^2 =$ 4.60, $P\langle$ 0.05) and also their relapse rates ($X^2 =$ 6.59, $P\langle$ 0.05). Therefore, *Xiao Chai Hu Tang* is obviously more effective than chlorpheniramine.

IgA levels found in the nasal secretions in the treatment group were 1.59 plus or minus 2.06gh before treatment and 3.85 plus or minus 2.84gh after treatment. This was compared to IgA levels in 65 healthy persons which were 2.35 plus or minus 2.75gh. Therefore, IgA levels were markedly low before treatment in the allergic rhinitis group and had significantly risen in the same group after treatment with *Xiao Chai Hu Tang*. IgE levels in the nasal secretions in the treatment group were 63.54 plus or minus 46.50Iu/ml before treatment and 30.23 plus or minus 29,10Iu/ml after treatment. Hence *Xiao Chai Hu Tang* significantly lowered IgE levels in their nasal secretions.

Discussion:

According to the authors, allergic rhinitis is due to spleen/lung qi vacuity, insecurity of the defensive exterior, and loose interstices. Thus wind cold takes advantage of vacuity and enters, assailing and harassing the nasal cavity. Hence the main branch symptoms are nasal itching, sneezing, clear mucus runny nose, and nasal obstruction. According to Japanese research reported by Zhang

Zhi-jun in issue #10, 1993 of the *Zhong Yi Za Zhi (Journal of Chinese Medicine)*, *Xiao Chai Hu Tang* has relatively strong anti-allergy, anti-inflammatory, and strengthening the immune function abilities. Therefore it can treat both the branch and the root simultaneously. Within this formula, Bupleurum clears heat and resolves the exterior. Hence, exterior evils obtain diffusion to the outside. Scutellaria clears heat and dries dampness. When combined with Bupleurum, they externally percolate and internally clear, expel cold and remove evils. Ginseng and Red Dates open the network vessels and quicken the blood, fortify the spleen and supplement the qi, support the righteous and dispel evils, and protect against evils being transmitted internally. Uncooked Ginger and Licorice regulate cold and heat, harmonize the constructive and defensive, clear heat, resolve toxins, and open the portals. According to modern medical theory, Bupleurum, Scutellaria, Ginseng, Licorice, uncooked Ginger, and Red Dates are antipyretic, antimicrobial, anti-inflammatory, and anti-allergic and increase the body's immune function. They also improve microcirculation, increasing the volume of blood flow, while decreasing inflammatory reactions affecting the capillaries. Typically, after administering this formula for two weeks, nasal itching, sneezing, clear runny nose, and nasal obstruction were all markedly diminished and the inflammatory reactions of the nasal cavity obviously had disappeared. Since the effectiveness rate is high, the recurrence rate is low, there is no particular toxicity, and both root and branch are treated simultaneously, *Xiao Chai Hu Tang* is an effective formula for the treatment of allergic rhinitis.

From "The Treatment of Allergic Rhinitis Mainly by Moxibustion" by Zhang Gui-rong *et al.*, *Zhong Guo Zhen Jiu (Chinese National Acupuncture & Moxibustion)*, #4, 1995, p. 55

There were 135 patients in this clinical audit. Of these, 75 were men and 60 were women. They ranged in age from as young as 7 to as old as 58. However, the majority of these patients were under 20 years old. The disease course was as short as 4 months to as long as 20 years. Treatment lasted from 10-40 days.

Treatment method:

The points chosen consisted of: *Yin Tang* (M-HN-3), *Zu San Li* (St 36), *He Gu* (LI 4), *Fei Shu* (Bl 13). These were treated by indirect moxibustion on top of slices of uncooked Rhizoma Zingiberis (*Jiang Pian*). These were cut as thick as a coin and a needle was used to poke holes in these. Each point was moxaed with 3 cones until the skin was flushed red. The points were treated 1 time each day with 10 days equaling 1 course of treatment. Chinese medicinals consisted of: Wine (stir-fried) Radix Scutellariae Baicalensis (*Jiu Qin*), Rhizoma Atractylodis (*Cang Zhu*), Rhizoma Pinelliae Ternatae (*Ban Xia*), Flos Magnoliae Liliflorae (*Xin Yi*), Radix Ligustici Wallichii (*Chuan Xiong*), Radix Angelicae Dahuricae (*Bai Zhi*), Gypsum Fibrosum (*Shi Gao*), Radix Panacis Ginseng (*Ren Shen*), Radix Puerariae (*Ge Gen*). One *ji* of these was decocted in water and administered each day with a continuous administration of seven days.

Definition of treatment outcomes:

Cure meant that the clinical symptoms completely disappeared and one year later there had been no recurrence. Fair or good effect meant that the greater part of the clinical symptoms had disappeared and, although there was recurrence, the symptoms were reduced. No effect meant that there was no change in the clinical symptoms.

Treatment outcomes:

Based on the above definitions, of these 135 patients, 89 (65.9%) were cured, 44 (32.6%) got a fair or good effect, and two (1.5%) experienced no effect. Thus the total effectiveness rate was 98.5%.

Case history:

The patient was a 21 year-old female. She came for her initial examination on Oct. 16, 1992. For five years she'd had nasal congestion, nasal itching, and clear runny nose. Her symptoms were worse in the fall and winter. However, she sometimes did have occurrences in the spring and summer. She was diagnosed as suffering from allergic rhinitis. She received moxibustion combined with the internal administration of Chinese medicinals. After five times, her nasal itching had disappeared, the flow of qi through both nostrils was free and fine, and the runny nose had markedly diminished. She received a total of seven *ji* and two courses of moxibustion. After that, her symptoms completely disappeared and there was no recurrence on follow-up after one year.

From "The Treatment of 120 Cases of Allergic Rhinitis with *Suo Quan Wan Jia Jian* (Withdraw the Spring Pills with Additions & Subtractions)" by Chen De-jiang, *Yun Nan Zhong Yi Zhong Yao Za Zhi (Yunnan Journal of Chinese Medicine & Chinese Medicinals)*, #5, 1955, p. 45-46

Suo Quan Wan is from the *Fu Ren Liang Fang (Fine Formulas for Women)*. It is composed of Fructus Alpiniae Oxyphyllae (*Yi Zhi Ren*), Radix Dioscoreae Oppositae (*Huai Shan Yao*), and Radix Linderae Strychnifoliae (*Wu Yao*). Its function is to warm the kidneys and secure and astringe. It mainly treats lower source vacuity chill leading to frequent, numerous urination and pediatric incontinence. Based on this clinical experience, the author has used this formula with modifications to treat 120 cases of allergic rhinitis with very good results.

Of these 120 patients, 50 were men and 70 were women. Their ages ranged from as young as 17 to as old as 45. The course of their disease had lasted from a minimum of one month to a maximum of four years. All these patients had been examined in the ear, nose, and throat department.

Treatment method:

The formula consisted of Fructus Alpiniae Oxyphyllae (*Yi Zhi Ren*), 15g, Radix Dioscoreae Oppositae (*Shan Yao*), 12g, Radix Linderae Strychnifoliae (*Wu Yao*), 10g, Radix Astragali Membranacei (*Huang Qi*), 15g, Rhizoma Atractylodis (*Cang Zhu*), 10g, Fructus Xanthii Sibirici (*Cang Er Zi*), 10g, Herba Cum Radice Asari Seiboldi (*Xi Xin*), 3g, Flos Magnoliae Liliflorae (*Xin Yi*), 10g, Fructus Pruni Mume (*Wu Mei*), 15g, Fructus Schizandrae Chinensis (*Wu Wei Zi*), 15g, Radix Ledebouriellae Divaricatae (*Fang Feng*), 6g, Radix Glycyrrhizae (*Gan Cao*), 3g. One *ji* was decocted and administered each day. A high fire was used and these medicinals were decocted two times. The first decoction was for 25 minutes and the second for 15 minutes. Both decoctions resulted in a combined volume of liquid of approximately 300ml. This was divided into 2 doses and administered on an empty stomach in the morning and evening.

Treatment outcomes:

Of the 120 cases, after treatment, the clinical symptoms disappeared and did not return within six months in 80 cases who were thus considered cured. In another 40 cases, the greater portion of their clinical symptoms disappeared. However, they recurred within 3 months. In these cases, the protocol was considered to be markedly effective. Thus the total effectiveness rate was 100%.

Discussion:

The *Nei Jing (Inner Classic)* says, "The lungs rule the snivel." "Difficulty 40" of the *Nan Jing (Classic of Difficulties)* says, "The lungs rule fluids." Snivel is one of the five fluids, and the five fluids are ruled by the kidneys. If the kidneys are vacuous, they do not store. Thus fluids and humors are discharged externally from the portal of the nose to become snivel. Therefore, treatment should warm the kidneys and secure and astringe. This is why the author has chosen *Suo Quan Wan*. In addition, the lungs open into the portal of the nose. The lungs (metal) are the mother of the kidneys (water), and it is said, "If there is vacuity, supplement the mother."

Thus it is appropriate to supplement the lungs and boost the qi, diffuse and free the flow of the portals of the nose. Hence the use of Alpinia, Dioscorea, and Astragalus treats the root. Xanthium and Flos Magnoliae free the flow of the portals of the nose; Atractylodes and Asarum dry dampness, warm the lungs, and transform rheum; while sour-flavored Mume and Schizandra restrain, astringe, and secure fluids and humors; thus treating the root. The lungs and kidneys are treated together, branch and root are simultaneously addressed, and therefore a good effect is experienced.

Case Histories

In order to help readers get a better feel for how Chinese medicine treats respiratory allergies, I have given below some more case histories. These are the stories of real-life people who have been treated with acupuncture and/or Chinese medicine for allergic rhinitis and asthma and gotten a good effect. Hopefully, you will be able to see yourself and your symptoms in these stories and be encouraged to give acupuncture and Chinese medicine a try.

Case 1.

The patient was a 70 year-old retired woman. Her major complaint was allergic rhinitis and asthma for more than 60 years. When her allergies flared up in the spring and fall or when she was around dogs and cats, itchy eyes and runny nose soon turned into asthmatic wheezing. If this continued for more than a day, she would then develop sinusitis. At the time of her first visit, the patient had a cough with copious white mucus. She had difficulty lying down and a tight chest. Clear, watery mucus flowed from her nose and her eyes were red and itchy.

In addition, she had heart palpitations, trouble going to sleep, and was easily awoken during the night. She got up to urinate three to four times each night. Her hands and feet were cold, her ankles were slightly edematous, and she caught cold easily. Her appetite and energy were both low, with two to three bowel movements per day. The stools themselves tended to be dry. She was currently being medicated with Proventrilo, Theodur, Prednisone, and

Synthroid. Her tongue was red with a deep crack running down the center with thick, white fur which was peeled in some areas. Her pulse was surging, slippery, and rapid. Her Western medical diagnosis was allergic rhinitis and asthma with recurrent sinusitis.

Based on the above signs and symptoms, this woman's Chinese medical pattern discrimination was a (spleen) qi and (kidney) yin vacuity with phlegm dampness obstructing her lungs. The treatment principles for this pattern are to fortify the spleen and supplement the qi, supplement the kidneys and enrich yin, transform phlegm, eliminate dampness, and loosen the chest. Therefore, the patient was given acupuncture at:

Ying Xiang (LI 20) for the runny nose
Zan Zhu (Bl 2) for the itchy eyes
Tai Yuan (Lu 9) for the lungs
Tai Xi (Ki 3) for the kidneys
San Yin Jiao (Sp 6) for the spleen and kidneys
Zu San Li (St 36) for the stomach and, therefore, the spleen
Feng Long (St 40) for phlegm dampness
Shan Zhong (CV 17) to loosen the chest
Fei Shu (Bl 13) for the lungs
Pi Shu (Bl 20) for the spleen
Shen Shu (Bl 23) for the kidneys

At the same time, she was prescribed two packets of Chinese herbs:

Radix Pseudostellariae (*Tai Zi Shen*), 9g
Fructus Schisandrae Chinensis (*Wu Wei Zi*), 6g
Tube Ophiopogonis Japonici (*Mai Men Dong*), 9g
Sclerotium Poriae Cocos (*Yun Fu Ling*), 12g
Rhizoma Dioscoreae Oppositae (*Huai Shan Yao*), 9g
Semen Pruni Armeniacae (*Ku Xing Ren*), 9g
Cortex Radicis Mori Albi (*Sang Bai Pi*), 9g
Folium Eriobotryae Japonicae (*Pi Pa Ye*), 9g
Semen Raphani Sativi (*Lai Fu Zi*), 6g
mix-fried Radix Glycyrrhizae (*Zhi Gan Cao*), 6g

In addition to the above Chinese herbs and acupuncture, the patient was advised to eat a clear, bland diet of cooked, not raw foods. In particular, she was instructed to stay away from sugars and sweets, dairy products and especially yogurt and cheese, fruit juices, tomatoes and tomato sauce, peanuts and peanut butter, and wheat as much as possible. She was also asked to particularly stay away from yeasted bread. Further, the patient was taught how to do Chinese self-massage every day.

Two days later, the patient reported that her runny nose and itchy eyes had cleared up. She was surprised that her allergies had not developed into sinusitis. Her cough and the amount of phlegm in her lungs was decreased, but her chest was still tight and she still was able to cough up phlegm in the morning. Her energy was still low, but her appetite was better. Her tongue was red with peeled fur, and her pulse was now bowstring and rapid. Therefore, it was decided to continue with basically the same Chinese herbal formula but to increase the ingredients for transforming phlegm and to add some ingredients for clearing heat from the liver. Thus the prescription now read:

Folium Mori Albi (*Sang Ye*), 9g
Cortex Radicis Mori Albi (*Sang Bai Pi)*, 9g
Flos Chrysanthemi Morifolii (*Ju Hua*), 9g
Tuber Ophiopogonis Japonici (*Mai Dong*), 9g
Radix Glehniae Littoralis (*Sha Shen*), 9g
Sclerotium Poriae Cocos (*Fu* Ling), 12g
Semen Pruni Armeniacae (*Xing Ren*), 9g
Bulbus Fritillariae Cirrhosae (*Chuan Bei Mu*), 9g
Pericarpium Trichosanthis Kirlowii (*Gua Lou Pi*), 9g
Radix Glycyrrhizae (*Gan Cao*), 6g

The patient was given eight days supply of this formula. At the same time, she received another acupuncture formula in order to boost her qi, transform phlegm, and loosen her chest as well as clear heat from her liver. The points needled consisted of:

113

Tai Chong (Liv 3) to course the liver and resolve depression
He Gu (LI 4) to clear heat
Qu Chi (LI 11) to clear heat
San Yin Jiao (Sp 6) to supplement the spleen and kidneys
Lie Que (Lu 7) to diffuse the lungs
Zu San Li (St 36) to supplement the spleen via the stomach
Shan Zhong (CV 17) to loosen the chest
Fei Shu (Bl 13) for the lungs
Pi Shu (Bl 20) for the spleen
Shen Shu (Bl 23) for the kidneys

After one week, the patient reported that she was breathing much better. Her chest did not feel so tight, she was able to lie down and breathe easily, and her energy was better. She was able to sleep better and she was only getting up one time per night to urinate. She was adhering to the clear, bland diet quite well and she enjoyed doing the Chinese self-massage every day. Because she was over any acute attacks, she was taught how to do moxibustion in order to strengthen her spleen and kidneys. She was given several Chinese medicinal porridge recipes to include in her regular diet, and a Chinese herbal prescription was written for more long-term root treatment. This prescription was filled in the form of desiccated, powdered extracts which do not require cooking but are simply mixed with boiled water and drunk three times per day. The Chinese herbal prescription was called *Chang Shou Ba Wei Wan Jia Wei* (Long Life Eight Flavors Pills with Added Flavors). It consisted of:

Tuber Ophiopogonis Japonici (*Mai Dong*), 12g
Fructus Schisandrae Chinensis (*Wu Wei Zi*), 9g
cooked Radix Rehmanniae (*Shu Di*), 12g
Radix Dioscoreae Oppositae (*Shan Yao*), 9g
Fructus Cornus Officinalis (*Shan Zhu Yu*), 9g
Sclerotium Poriae Cocos (*Fu Ling*), 9g
Cortex Radicis Moutan (*Dan Pi*), 9g
Rhizoma Alismatis (*Ze Xie*), 9g
Bulbus Fritillariae Cirrhosae (*Chuan Bei Mu*), 9g

Radix Polygalae Tenuifoliae (*Yuan Zhi*), 9g
mix-fried Radix Astragali Membranacei (*Huang Qi*), 15g
Cordyceps Sinensis (*Dong Chong Xia Cao*), 6g

The woman continued on this formula for six months. On follow-up after one year, she had not had any allergic episodes and no asthma attacks. She was not getting up to urinate at night, and she felt 10 years younger than her former self. Her doctor had taken her off all her Western medications except for the Synthroid.

Case 2.

The patient was a 10 year-old boy. He experienced bad hay-fever each spring. When he was around cats, dogs, rabbits, or horses, he developed asthma. He also had a tendency to recurrent tonsillitis in the fall and winter. His MD had not suggested a tonsillectomy yet, but each winter, the child was on antibiotics at least a couple of times. He had been taking antibiotics off and on since he was seven months old when he had developed recurrent earaches. At the moment, he had a copiously runny nose, sneezing and nasal congestion, red eyes, itchy eyes, throat, and nose, and pronounced irritability. The child was slightly overweight, and the mother reported that he drank lots of orange juice, ate lots of ice cream, cookies, and chocolate, and had a craving for bread. His tongue was fat and enlarged with the marks of his teeth on the borders of the tongue. The tongue fur was white and slightly slimy. His pulse was bowstring and slippery overall while being floating and fine in the right bar position (associated with the spleen) and floating and slippery in the right inch position (associated with the lungs).

This child's Chinese pattern discrimination was external invasion by wind evils with spleen vacuity, liver depression transforming heat, and phlegm dampness. The treatment principles were to resolve the exterior and dispel wind, supplement the spleen and eliminate dampness, course and clear the liver and open the portals (of the nose). Because the child was "needle shy", he was treated with seven star hammering. This was tapped all along the back of his neck, his temples, and all around the sides of his nose. In addition, *He Gu* (LI 4) and *Tai Chong* (Liv 3) were tapped to resolve the exterior and course the liver, as was *Feng Long* (St 40) in order to help transform phlegm. His mother then did seven star hammering every day for the next five days. At the same time, he was prescribed the following Chinese herbal formula:

Radix Astragali Membranacei (*Huang Qi*), 9g
Radix Panacis Ginseng (*Ren Shen*),4.5g
Rhizoma Atractylodis Macrocephalae (*Bai Zhu*), 6g
Rhizoma Pinelliae Ternatae (*Ban Xia*), 6g
Pericarpium Citri Reticulatae (*Chen Pi*), 6g
Sclerotium Poriae Cocos (*Fu Ling*), 9g
mix-fried Radix Glycyrrhizae (*Gan Cao*), 4.5g
Radix Angelicae Sinensis (*Dang Gui*), 3g
Radix Schisandrae Chinensis (*Wu Wei Zi*), 6g
Herba Asari Cum Radice (*Xi Xin*), 1.5g
Radix Bupleuri (*Chai Hu*), 6g
Rhizoma Cimicifugae (*Sheng Ma*), 6g
Flos Chrysanthemi Morifolii (*Ju Hua*), 6g
Fructus Xanthii Sibirici (*Cang Er Zi*), 6g
Flos Magnoliae Liliflorae (*Xin Yi Hua*), 6g

This prescription was administered for one week, at the end of which time, the hay fever had disappeared. The child's mother was instructed on the clear, bland diet, and she promised to do her best in getting her child to stick to this. This was in the spring, and the child had no more hay fever that season. In the fall, he was prescribed a modification of *Xiao Chai Hu Tang* (Minor Bupleurum Decoction) in desiccated, powdered extract form. This consisted of:

Radix Bupleuri (*Chai Hu*), 6g
Radix Panacis Ginseng (*Ren Shen*), 4.5g
Radix Scutellariae Baicalensis (*Huang Qin*), 6g

Rhizoma Pinelliae Ternatae (*Ban Xia*), 6g
Pericarpium Citri Reticulatae (*Chen Pi*), 6g
Sclerotium Poriae Cocos (*Fu Ling*), 9g
mix-fried Radix Glycyrrhizae (*Gan Cao*), 3g
Fructus Zizyphi Jujubae (*Da Zao*), 3 pieces
uncooked Rhizoma Zingiberis (*Sheng Jiang*), 2 slices

This was given from September through April. The child never caught a cold that year, did not have tonsillitis, did not have any hay fever in the spring, and did not miss a single day of school that year.

According to Chinese medicine, antibiotics are excessively "bitter and cold" and can damage the spleen. Although their use is sometimes warranted, they are often over- or unnecessarily prescribed. When over- or unnecessarily prescribed, although they do eliminate inflammation due to bacterial infection, they can also weaken the spleen. Since the spleen is the root of qi and blood production, including the defensive qi, damage of the spleen typically results in a defensive qi vacuity. This leaves the person open to easy attack as external wind evils take advantage of this vacuity to enter and cause disease. Therefore, it is not uncommon to see recurrent infections followed by repeated courses of antibiotics. In this case, the repeated antibiotics weaken and further weaken the spleen. Thus the person is repeatedly invaded by wind evils. In such cases, it is extremely important to break this cycle by going without antibiotics unless absolutely necessary. As long as antibiotics are given again and again, the person's spleen has little chance of recuperating.

In addition, in this case, we see that the child has a long history of complaints beginning in infancy. While these may be diagnosed as different diseases in Western medicine, Chinese doctors see these as a continuum, certain diseases occurring at certain ages, however all due to spleen vacuity with accumulation of phlegm and dampness. For more information on Chinese medicine and children's diseases, see my *Keeping Your Child Healthy with Chinese Medicine* also published by Blue Poppy Press.

Case 3.

The patient was a 43 year-old female airline pilot. She said her hormones were "on a rampage" and that she was having allergic reactions to many things. When asked what these things were, she said dogs and cats. She had been allergic to these younger in her life but then had "outgrown" them. Now they were coming back, with coughing and red, painful, itchy eyes. The cough was dry, occasionally there was wheezing, and her chest felt tight. She had a skin rash on her inner arms. It had previously been made up of many small blisters. Now it was a diffuse red rash which was very itchy. Her menstruation had come recently four days late instead of several days early. She complained that her eyes were always irritated and out of focus. She had continuous headaches right behind her eyes and occasionally in the middle of the back of her head. Her memory was "off" and her focus was not good. Her bowel movements were OK, but her appetite was decreased. Nonetheless, she had gained six pounds in the last year. Her energy was good in the morning but then"crashed" at 3 PM and she was in bed by 9 PM. She slept "like a rock." In addition, she had severe low back pain, her feet were always cold, and she had zero libido.

The patient's tongue was light red, swollen, had the marks of her teeth on its edges, was darker all around its rim, and had thin, white fur. Her pulse was floating and slippery in the right inch position (associated with the lungs), bowstring and floating in the right bar (associated with the spleen), and fine, bowstring, and not very forceful in the right cubit (associated with kidney yang). On the left, the inch (associated with the heart) was floating vacuous, the bar (associated with the liver) was bowstring, and the cubit (associated with kidney yin) was fine, a little bowstring, and less forceful than the right cubit.

118

All this adds up to the following Chinese pattern discrimination: depressive heat in the liver and lungs damaging fluids, spleen vacuity, and kidney yang vacuity. The treatment principles were to resolve depression and clear the liver and lungs, fortify the spleen and boost the qi, and invigorate the kidneys and strengthen the low back. In addition, because it was day 17 in her menstrual cycle, the principles of quickening the blood and regulating menstruation were also used. Because the woman lived 2,000 miles away, a formula was written but no acupuncture was given. The formula consisted of:

Radix Bupleuri (*Chai Hu*), 9g
Radix Astragali Membranacei (*Huang Qi*), 18g
Radix Codonopsitis Pilosulae (*Dang Shen*), 9g
Radix Dioscoreae Oppositae (*Shan Yao*), 9g
Sclerotium Poriae Cocos (*Fu Ling*), 9g
Tuber Ophiopogonis Japonici (*Mai Dong*), 12g
Radix Scutellariae Baicalensis (*Huang Qin*), 12g
Fructus Gardeniae Jasminoidis (*Shan Zhi Zi*), 9g
Flos Chrysanthemi Morifolii (*Ju Hua*), 9g
Radix Rubrus Paeoniae Lactiflorae (*Chi Shao*), 9g
Radix Ligustici Wallichii (*Chuan Xiong*), 15g
Radix Angelicae Sinensis (*Dang Gui*), 9g
uncooked Radix Rehmanniae (*Sheng Di*), 12g
Cortex Eucommiae Ulmoidis (*Du Zhong*), 9g
Radix Dipsaci (*Xu Duan*), 9g
mix-fried Radix Glycyrrhizae (*Gan Cao*), 6g
Fructus Zizyphi Jujubae (*Da Zao*), 3 pieces
uncooked Rhizoma Zingiberis (*Sheng Jiang*), 3 slices

This formula was prescribed for three days. At the end of this time, the patient called to say that the headaches were gone, her eyes were slightly clearer, and her skin had no red bumps. However, her skin still itched. Therefore, her formula was rewritten to include Fructus Tribuli Terrestris (*Bai Ji Li*), 15g, for the itching, while the Red Dates and Ginger were subtracted as being essentially superfluous.

119

After 10 days, the patient called in again. Now she said that everything was definitely better. Her menstruation had come on time and the blood was much less clotty. Her low back was good. However, her skin still itched and she had lots of gas each time she drank the herbs. Therefore, her prescription was again rewritten in order to make it more effective without *any* side effects:

Radix Astragali Membranacei (*Huang Qi*), 18g
cooked Radix Rehmanniae (*Shu Di*), 12g
Radix Angelicae Sinensis (*Dang Gui*), 9g
Radix Dioscoreae Oppositae (*Shan Yao*), 15g
Fructus Corni Officinalis (*Shan Zhu Yu*), 9g
Sclerotium Poriae Cocos (*Fu Ling*), 9g
Cortex Radicis Moutan (*Dan Pi*), 9g
Flos Chrysanthemi Morifollii (*Ju Hua*), 9g
Radix Scutellariae Baicalensis (*Huang Qin*), 9g
Tuber Ophiopogonis Japonici (*Mai Dong*), 12g
Fructus Tribuli Terrestris (*Bai Ji Li*), 15g
Bombyx Batryticatus (*Jiang Can*), 9g
Radix Ledebouriellae Divaricatae (*Fang Feng*), 9g
Herba Seu Flos Schizonepetae Tenuifoliae (*Jing Jie*), 9g

These modifications were meant to reduce the abdominal bloating when taking these herbs at the same time more effectively eliminate the skin itching. At the end of another two weeks, the patient reported that all her symptoms had been eliminated and that she felt great!

Finding a Professional Practitioner of Chinese Medicine

Traditional Chinese medicine is one of the fastest growing holistic health care systems in the West today. At the present time, there are 50 colleges in the United States alone which offer 3-4 year training programs in acupuncture, moxibustion, Chinese herbal medicine, and Chinese medical massage. In addition, many of the graduates of these programs have done postgraduate studies at colleges and hospitals in China, Taiwan, Hong Kong, and Japan. Further, a growing number of trained Oriental medical practitioners have immigrated from China, Japan, and Korea to practice acupuncture and Chinese herbal medicine in the West.

Traditional Chinese medicine, including acupuncture, is a discreet and independent health care profession. It is not simply a modality that can easily be added to the array of techniques of some other health care profession. The study of Chinese medicine, acupuncture, and Chinese herbs is as rigorous as is the study of allopathic, chiropractic, naturopathic, or homeopathic medicines. Previous training in any one of these other systems does not automatically confer competence or knowledge in Chinese medicine. In order to get the full benefits and safety of Chinese medicine, one should seek out professionally trained and credentialed practitioners.

In the United States, recognition that acupuncture and Chinese medicine are their own independent professions has led to the creation of the National Commission for the Certification of Acupuncture & Oriental Medicine (NCCAOM). This commission has created and administers a national board examination in both acupuncture and Chinese herbal medicine in order to insure minimum levels of professional competence and safety. Those who pass the acupuncture exam append the letters Dipl. Ac. (Diplomate of Acupuncture) after their names, while those who pass the Chinese herbal exam use the letters Dipl. C.H. (Diplomate of Chinese Herbs). I recommend that persons wishing to experience the benefits of acupuncture and Chinese medicine should seek treatment in the U.S. *only* from those who are NCCAOM certified.

In addition, in the United States, acupuncture is a legal, independent health care profession in more than half the states. A few other states require acupuncturists to work under the supervision of MDs, while in a number of states, acupuncture has yet to receive legal status. In states where acupuncture is licensed and regulated, the names of acupuncture practitioners can be found in the *Yellow Pages* of your local phone book or through contacting your State Department of Health, Board of Medical Examiners, or Department of Regulatory Agencies. In states without licensure, it is doubly important to seek treatment only from NCCAOM diplomates.

When seeking a qualified and knowledgeable practitioner, word of mouth referrals are important. Satisfied patients are the most reliable credential a practitioner can have. It is appropriate to ask the practitioner for references from previous patients treated for the same problem. It is best to work with a practitioner who communicates effectively enough for the patient to feel understood and for the Chinese medical diagnosis and treatment plan to make sense. In all cases, a professional practitioner of Chinese medicine should be able *and willing* to give a written traditional Chinese diagnosis of the patient's pattern upon request.

For further information regarding the practice of Chinese medicine and acupuncture in the United States of America and for referrals to local professional associations and practitioners in the United States, prospective patients may contact:

The National Commission for the Certification of Acupuncture & Oriental Medicine
P.O. Box 97075
Washington, DC 20090-7075
Tel: (202) 232-1404
Fax: (202) 462-6157

The National Acupuncture & Oriental Medicine Alliance
14637 Starr Rd., SE
Olalla, WA 98357
Tel: (206) 851-6895
Fax: (206) 728-4841
E mail: 76143.2061@compuserve.com

The American Association of Oriental Medicine
433 Front St.
Catasauqua, PA 18032-2506
Tel: (610) 433-2448
Fax: (610) 433-1832

Learning More About Chinese Medicine

For more information on Chinese medicine in general, see:

The Web That Has No Weaver: Understanding Chinese Medicine by Ted Kaptchuk, Congdon & Weed, NY, 1983. This is the best overall introduction to Chinese medicine for the serious lay reader. It has been a standard since it was first published over a dozen years ago and it has yet to be replaced.

Chinese Secrets of Health & Longevity by Bob Flaws, Sound True, Boulder, CO, 1996. This is a six tape audio cassette course introducing Chinese medicine to laypeople. It covers basic Chinese medical theory, Chinese dietary therapy, Chinese herbal medicine, acupuncture, *qi gong*, *feng shui*, deep relaxation, lifestyle, and more.

Fundamentals of Chinese Medicine by the East Asian Medical Studies Society, Paradigm Publications, Brookline, MA, 1985. This is a more technical introduction and overview of Chinese medicine intended for professional entry level students.

Traditional Medicine in Contemporary China by Nathan Sivin, Center for Chinese Studies, University of Michigan, Ann Arbor, 1987. This book discusses the development of Chinese medicine in China in the last half century.

Imperial Secrets of Health and Longevity by Bob Flaws, Blue Poppy Press, Boulder, CO, 1994. This book includes a section on

Chinese dietary therapy and generally introduces the basic concepts of good health according to Chinese medicine.

Chinese Herbal Remedies by Albert Y. Leung, Universe Books, NY, 1984. This book is about simple Chinese herbal home remedies.

Legendary Chinese Healing Herbs by Henry C. Lu, Sterling Publishing, Inc., NY, 1991. This book is a fun way to begin learning about Chinese herbal medicine. It is full of interesting and entertaining anecdotes about Chinese medicinal herbs.

The Mystery of Longevity by Liu Zheng-cai, Foreign Languages Press, Beijing, 1990. This book is also about general principles and practice promoting good health according to Chinese medicine.

For more information on Chinese dietary therapy, see:

The Dao of Healthy Eating According to Traditional Chinese Medicine by Bob Flaws, Blue Poppy Press, Inc., Boulder, CO, 1997. This book is a layperson's primer on Chinese dietary therapy. It includes detailed sections on the clear, bland diet as well as sections on chronic candidiasis, allergies, and much more.

Prince Wen Hui's Cook: Chinese Dietary Therapy by Bob Flaws & Honora Lee Wolfe, Paradigm Publications, Brookline, MA, 1983. This book is an introduction to Chinese dietary therapy. Although some of the information it contains is dated, it does give the Chinese medicinal descriptions of most foods commonly eaten in the West.

The Book of Jook: Chinese Medicinal Porridges, A Healthy Alternative to the Typical Western Breakfast by Bob Flaws, Blue Poppy Press, Inc., Boulder, CO, 1995. This book is specifically about Chinese medicinal porridges made with very simple combinations of Chinese medicinal herbs.

Chinese Medicinal Wines & Elixirs by Bob Flaws, Blue Poppy Press, Inc., Boulder, CO, 1995. This book is a large collection of simple, one, two, and three ingredient Chinese medicinal wines which can be made at home.

Chinese Medicinal Teas: Simple, Proven Folk Formulas for Treating Disease & Promoting Health by Zong Xiao-fan & Gary Liscum, Blue Poppy Press, Inc., Boulder, CO, 1997. Like the above two books, this book is about one, two, and three ingredient Chinese medicinal teas which are easy to make and can be used at home as adjuncts to other, professionally prescribed treatments or for the promotion of health and prevention of disease.

The Tao of Nutrition by Maoshing Ni, Union of Tao and Man, Los Angeles, 1989

Harmony Rules: The Chinese Way of Health Through Food by Gary Butt & Frena Bloomfield, Samuel Weiser, Inc., York Beach, ME, 1985

Chinese System of Food Cures: Prevention & Remedies by Henry C. Lu, Sterling Publishing Co., NY, 1986

A Practical English-Chinese Library of Traditional Chinese Medicine: Chinese Medicated Diet ed. by Zhang En-qin, Shanghai College of Traditional Chinese Medicine Publishing House, Shanghai, 1990

Eating Your Way to Health — Dietotherapy in Traditional Chinese Medicine by Cai Jing-feng, Foreign Languages Press, Beijing, 1988

Qi gong:

Qi gong is the modern generic name for any of thousands of different Chinese health exercises. Typically, *qi gong* exercises combine various proportions of meditative concentration, visualization, deep relaxation, breath patterns, and rhythmic physical movements. Although I have not been able to find any specific *qi gong* exercises for respiratory allergies, certainly *qi gong* can strengthen the qi of the entire body, including the defensive qi, as well as specifically supplementing the qi of the lungs, spleen, and kidneys. Therefore, readers interested in learning about Chinese health exercises and how these may fit into a total health and healing regime should see the following books.

Chi Kung: Cultivating Personal Energy by James MacRitchie, Element, Shaftesbury, UK, 1993. This is a short, well-written introduction to *qi gong*. It includes the history and theory of *qi gong* as well as a selection of different *qi gong* exercises.

The Chinese Exercise Book by Dahong Zhou, Hartley & Marks, Pt. Roberts, WA, 1984. This book teaches several of the most famous systems of *qi gong*.

Exercises Illustrated: Ancient Way to Keep Fit by Zong Wu & Li Mao, Shelter Publications, Inc., Bolinas, CA, 1992. This is a very beautiful book filled with ancient and modern Chinese drawings and paintings of various *qi gong* exercises.

Change the Picture: A Qigong Workbook by Yu-cheng Huang, Ching Ying Tai Chi Kung Fu Association, Chicago, IL. This book presents a systematic, progressive regimen for learning *qi gong*. Theory and method are provided in a series of self-study lessons allowing the student to increase their understanding and ability with *qi gong* through practice of a series of well-illustrated exercises designed to learn to feel the qi, lead the qi, supplement the qi, etc.

Knocking At the Gate of Life by Edward C. Chang, Rodale Press Inc., Emmaus, PA. This book presents *qi gong* exercises for hundreds of different health problems.

Qigong / Chi Kung: Awakening and Mastering the Medicine Within You by Roger Jahnke, Health Action, Santa Barbara, CA, undated. This is an excellent videotape for learning to do *qi gong*. A number of very simple yet effective exercises are given designed to improve health and treat disease.

Qigong: The Chinese Way of Health by Ken Cohen, Nederland, CO. This one hour videotape covers the two most basic forms of *qi gong*, the Six Healing Sounds and Standing Meditation. In particular, the Six Healing Sounds are particularly useful for treating disease due to dysfunction of the internal organs.

The Way of Qigong: The Art and Science of Chinese Energy Healing by Kenneth S. Cohen, Ballantine Books, NY, 1997. This book is, in my opinion, the single best book on *qi gong*. Although perhaps a little scholarly for some people's taste, this book presents the history of *qi gong*, explains the different types of *qi gong*, and includes basic guidelines for safe and effective *qi gong* practice.

Chinese Medical Glossary

Chinese medicine is a system unto itself. Its technical terms are uniquely its own and cannot be reduced to the definitions of Western medicine without destroying the very fabric and logic of Chinese medicine. Ultimately, because Chinese medicine was created in the Chinese language, Chinese medicine is best and really only understood in that language. Nevertheless, as Westerners trying to understand Chinese medicine, we must translate the technical terms of Chinese medicine in English words. If some of these technical translations sound at first peculiar and their meaning is not immediately transparent, this is because no equivalent concepts exist in everyday English.

In the past, some Western authors have erroneously translated technical Chinese medical terms using Western medical or at least quasi-scientific words in an attempt to make this system more acceptable to Western audiences. For instance, the words tonify and sedate are commonly seen in the Western Chinese medical literature even though, in the case of sedate, its meaning is 180° opposite to the Chinese understanding of the word *xie*. *Xie* means to drain off something which has pooled and accumulated. That accumulation is seen as something excess which should not be lingering where it is. Because it is accumulating somewhere where it shouldn't, it is impeding and obstructing whatever should be moving to and through that area. The word sedate comes from the Latin word *sedere*, to sit. Therefore, the word sedate means to make something sit still. In English, we get the word sediment from this same root. However, the Chinese *xie* means draining off that which is sitting somewhere erroneously.

Therefore, to think that one is going to sedate what is already sitting is a great mistake in understanding the clinical implication and application of this technical term.

Hence, in order to preserve the integrity of this system while still making it intelligible to English language readers, I have appended the following glossary of Chinese medical technical terms. The terms themselves are based on Nigel Wiseman's *English-Chinese Chinese-English Dictionary of Chinese Medicine* published by the Hunan Science & Technology Press in Changsha, People's Republic of China in 1995. Dr. Wiseman is, I believe, the greatest Western scholar in terms of the translation of Chinese medicine into English. As a Chinese reader myself, although I often find Wiseman's terms awkward sounding at first, I also think they convey most accurately the Chinese understanding and logic of these terms.

Acquired essence: Essence manufactured out of the surplus of qi and blood in turn created out of the refined essence of food and drink

Acupoints: Those places on the channels and network vessels where qi and blood tend to collect in denser concentrations, and thus those places where the qi and blood in the channels are especially available for manipulation

Acupuncture: The regulation of qi flow by the stimulation of certain points located on the channels and network vessels achieved mainly by insertion of fine needles into these points

Bedroom taxation: Fatigue or vacuity due to excessive sex

Blood: The red colored fluids which flow in the vessels and nourishes and constructs the tissues of the body

Blood stasis: Also called dead blood, malign blood, and dry blood, blood stasis is blood which is no longer moving through the vessels as it should. Instead it is precipitated in the vessels like silt in a river. Like silt, it then obstructs the free flow of the blood in the vessels and also impedes the production of new or fresh blood.

Blood vacuity: Insufficient blood manifesting in diminished nourishment, construction, and moistening of body tissues

Bowels: The hollow yang organs of Chinese medicine

Central qi: Also called the middle qi, this is synonymous with the spleen-stomach qi

Channels: The main routes for the distribution of qi and blood, but mainly qi

Clear: The pure or clear part of food and drink ingested which is then turned into qi and blood

Constructive qi: The qi which flows through the channels and nourishes and constructs the internal organs and body tissues

Counterflow: An erroneous flow of qi, usually upward but sometimes horizontally as well

Damp heat: A combination of accumulated dampness mixed with pathological heat often associated with sores, abnormal vaginal discharges, and some types of menstrual and body pain

Dampness: A pathological accumulation of body fluids

Decoction: A method of administering Chinese medicinals by boiling these medicinals in water, removing the dregs, and drinking the resulting medicinal liquid

Defensive qi: The yang qi which protects the exterior of the body from invasion by the environmental excesses

Depression: Stagnation and lack of movement, as in liver depression qi stagnation

Depressive heat: Heat due to enduring or severe qi stagnation which then transforms into heat

Drain: To drain off or away some pathological qi or substance from where it is replete or excess

Environmental excesses: A superabundance of wind, cold, dampness, dryness, heat, or summerheat in the external environment which can invade the body and cause disease

Essence: A stored, very potent form of substance and qi, usually yin when compared to yang qi, but can be transformed into yang qi

External causes of disease: The six environmental excesses

Five phase theory: An ancient Chinese system of correspondences dividing up all of reality into five phases which then mutually engender and check each other according to definite sequences

Heat toxins: A particularly virulent and concentrated type of pathological heat often associated with purulence (*i.e.*, pus formation), sores, and sometimes, but not always, malignancies

Impediment: A hindrance to the free flow of the qi and blood typically manifesting as pain and restriction in the range of movement of a joint or extremity

Internal causes of disease: The seven affects or emotions, namely, anger, joy (or excitement), sorrow, thought, fear, melancholy, and fright

Lassitude of the spirit: A listless of apathetic affect or emotional demeanor due to obvious fatigue of the mind and body

Life gate fire: Another name for kidney yang or kidney fire, seen as the ultimate source of yang qi in the body

Moxibustion: Burning the herb Artemisia Argyium on, over, or near acupuncture points in order to add yang qi, warm cold, or promote the movement of the qi and blood

Neither external nor internal causes of disease: A miscellaneous group of pathogenic factors including trauma, diet, overtaxation, insufficient exercise, poisoning, parasites, etc.

Network vessels: Small vessels which form a net-like web insuring the flow of qi and blood to all body tissues

Phlegm: A pathological accumulation of phlegm or mucus congealed from dampness or body fluids

Portals: Also called orifices, the openings of the sensory organs and the opening of the heart through which the spirit makes contact with the world outside

Qi: Activity, function, that which moves, transforms, defends, restrains, and warms

Qi mechanism: The process of transforming yin substance controlled and promoted by the qi, largely synonymous with the process of digestion

Qi vacuity: Insufficient qi manifesting in diminished movement, transformation, and function

Repletion: Excess or fullness, almost always pathological

Seven star hammer: A small hammer with needles embedded in its head used to stimulate acupoints without actually inserting needles

Spirit: The accumulation of qi in the heart which manifests as consciousness, sensory awareness, and mental-emotional function

Stagnation: Non-movement of the qi, lack of free flow, constraint

Supplement: To add to or augment, as in supplementing the qi, blood, yin, or yang

Turbid: The yin, impure, turbid part of food and drink which is sent downward to be excreted as waste

Vacuity: Emptiness or insufficiency, typically of qi, blood, yin, or yang

Vacuity cold: Obvious signs and symptoms of cold due to a lack or insufficiency of yang qi

Vacuity heat: Heat due to hyperactive yang in turn due to insufficient controlling yin

Vessels: The main routes for the distribution of qi and blood, but mainly blood

Viscera: The solid yin organs of Chinese medicine

Yang: In the body, function, movement, activity, transformation

Yang vacuity: Insufficient warming and transforming function giving rise to symptoms of cold in the body

Yin: In the body, substance and nourishment

Yin vacuity: Insufficient yin substance necessary to nourish, control, and counterbalance yang activity

Bibliography

Chinese language sources

Chu Zhen Zhi Liao Xue (A Study of Acupuncture Treatment), Li Zhong-yu, Sichuan Science & Technology Press, Chengdu, 1990

Han Ying Chang Yong Yi Xue Ci Hui (Chinese-English Glossary of Commonly Used Medical Terms), Huang Xiao-kai, People's Health & Hygiene Press, Beijing, 1982

Shang Hai Lao Zhong Yi Jing Yan Xuan Bian (A Selected Compilation of Shanghai Old Doctors' Experiences), Shanghai Science & Technology Press, Shanghai, 1984

Shi Yong Zhen Jiu Tui Na Zhi Liao Xue (A Study of Practical Acupuncture, Moxibustion & Tui Na Treatments), Xia Zhi-ping, Shanghai College of Chinese Medicine Press, Shanghai, 1990

Tan Zheng Lun (Treatise on Phlegm Conditions), Hou Tian-yin & Wang Chun-hua, People's Army Press, Beijing, 1989

Yi Zong Jin Jian (The Golden Mirror of Ancestral Medicine), Wu Qian *et al.*, People's Health & Hygiene Press, Beijing, 1985

Zhen Jiu Da Cheng (A Great Compendium of Acupuncture & Moxibustion), Yang Ji-zhou, People's Health & Hygiene Press, Beijing, 1983

Zhen Jiu Xue (A Study of Acupuncture & Moxibustion), Qiu Mao-liang *et al.*, Shanghai Science & Technology Press, Shanghai, 1985

Zhen Jiu Yi Xue (An Easy Study of Acupuncture & Moxibustion), Li Shou-xian, People's Health & Hygiene Press, Beijing, 1990

Zhong Guo Min Jian Cao Yao Fang (Chinese Folk Herbal Medicinal Formulas), Liu Guang-rui & Liu Shao-lin, Sichuan Science & Technology Press, Chengdu, 1992

Zhong Guo Zhen Jiu Chu Fang Xue (A Study of Chinese Acupuncture & Moxibustion Prescriptions), Xiao Shao-qing, Ningxia People's Press, Yinchuan, 1986

Zhong Guo Zhong Yi Mi Fang Da Quan (A Great Compendium of Chinese National Chinese Medical Secret Formulas), ed. by Hu Zhao-ming, Literary Propagation Publishing Company, Shanghai, 1992

Zhong Yi Hu Li Xue (A Study of Chinese Medical Nursing), Lu Su-ying, People's Health & Hygiene Press, Beijing, 1983

Zhong Yi Lin Chuang Ge Ke (Various Clinical Specialties in Chinese Medicine), Zhang En-qin *et al.*, Shanghai College of TCM Press, Shanghai, 1990

Zhong Yi Ling Yan Fang (Efficacious Chinese Medical Formulas), Lin Bin-zhi, Science & Technology Propagation Press, Beijing, 1991

English language sources

A Barefoot Doctor's Manual, revised & enlarged edition, Cloudburst Press, Mayne Isle, 1977

A Clinical Guide to Chinese Herbs and Formulae, Cheng Song-yu & Li Fei, Churchill & Livingstone, Edinburgh, 1993

A Compendium of TCM Patterns & Treatments, Bob Flaws & Daniel Finney, Blue Poppy Press, Boulder, CO, 1996

A Comprehensive Guide to Chinese Herbal Medicine, Chen Ze-lin & Chen Mei-fang, Oriental Healing Arts Institute, Long Beach, CA, 1992

A Glossary of Chinese Medical Terms & Acupuncture Points, Nigel Wiseman & Ken Boss, Paradigm Publications, Brookline, MA, 1990

The Dao of Healthy Eating According to Traditional Chinese Medicine, Bob Flaws, Blue Poppy Press, Boulder, CO, 1997

A Handbook of Differential Diagnosis with Key Signs & Symptoms, Therapeutic Principles, and Guiding Prescriptions, Ou-yang Yi, trans. by C. S. Cheung, Harmonious Sunshine Cultural Center, San Francisco, 1987

Chinese-English Terminology of Traditional Chinese Medicine, Shuai Xue-zhong *et al.*, Hunan Science & Technology Press, Changsha, 1983

Chinese-English Manual of Common-used Prescriptions in Traditional Chinese Medicine, Ou Ming, ed., Joint Publishing Co., Ltd., Hong Kong, 1989

Chinese Herbal Medicine: Formulas & Strategies, Dan Bensky & Randall Barolet, Eastland Press, Seattle, 1990

Chinese Herbal Medicine: Materia Medica, Dan Bensky & Andrew Gamble, second, revised edition, Eastland Press, Seattle, 1993

Chinese Medicinal Teas: Simple, Proven Folk Formulas for the Treatment of Disease and Promotion of Health, Zong Xiao-fan & Gary Liscum, Blue Poppy Press, Boulder, CO, 1997

Chinese Medicinal Wines & Elixirs, Bob Flaws, Blue Poppy Press, Boulder, CO, 1995

Chinese Self-massage Therapy, The Easy Way to Health, Fan Ya-li, Blue Poppy Press, Boulder, CO, 1996

Fundamentals of Chinese Acupuncture, Andrew Ellis, Nigel Wiseman & Ken Boss, Paradigm Publications, Brookline, MA, 1988

Fundamentals of Chinese Medicine, Nigel Wiseman & Andrew Ellis, Paradigm Publications, Brookline, MA, 1985

Handbook of Chinese Herbs and Formulas, Him-che Yeung, self-published, Los Angeles, 1985

In the Footsteps of the Yellow Emperor: Tracing the History of Traditional Acupuncture, Peter Eckman, Cypress Book Co., San Francisco, 1996

Knowing Practice: The Clinical Encounter of Chinese Medicine, Judith Farquhar, Westview Press, Boulder, CO, 1994

Medicine in China: A History of Ideas, Paul U. Unschuld, University of California Press, Berkeley, 1985

Oriental Materia Medica, A Concise Guide, Hong-yen Hsu, Oriental Healing Arts Institute, Long Beach, CA, 1986

Practical Traditional Chinese Medicine & Pharmacology: Clinical Experiences, Shang Xian-min *et al.*, New World Press, Beijing, 1990

Practical Traditional Chinese Medicine & Pharmacology: Herbal Formulas, Geng Jun-ying, *et al.*, New World Press, Beijing, 1991

Statements of Fact in Traditional Chinese Medicine, Bob Flaws, Blue Poppy Press, Boulder, CO, 1994

The Book of Jook: Chinese Medicinal Porridges, Bob Flaws, Blue Poppy Press, Boulder, CO, 1995

The Complete Book of Chinese Health and Healing, Daniel Reid, Shambhala, Boston, 1994

The English-Chinese Encyclopedia of Practical Traditional Chinese Medicine, Xuan Jia-sheng, ed., Higher Education Press, Beijing, 1990

The Essential Book of Traditional Chinese Medicine, Liu Yan-chi, trans. by Fang Ting-yu & Chen Lai-di, Columbia University Press, NY, 1988

The Merck Manual, 15th edition, ed. by Robert Berkow, Merck Sharp & Dohme Research Laboratories, Rahway, NJ, 1987

The Treatise on the Spleen & Stomach, Li Dong-yuan, trans. by Yang Shou-zhong, Blue Poppy Press, Boulder, CO, 1993

Traditional Medicine in Contemporary China, Nathan Sivin, University of Michigan, Ann Arbor, 1987

Zang Fu: The Organ Systems of Traditional Chinese Medicine, second edition, Jeremy Ross, Churchill Livingstone, Edinburgh, 1985

Index

145

OTHER BOOKS ON CHINESE MEDICINE AVAILABLE FROM BLUE POPPY PRESS

1775 Linden Ave, Boulder, CO 80304
For ordering 1-800-487-9296 PH. 303\447-8372 FAX 303\447-0740

A NEW AMERICAN ACUPUNC-TURE by Mark Seem, ISBN 0-936185-44-9

ACUPUNCTURE AND MOXI-BUSTION FORMULAS & TREAT-MENTS by Cheng Dan-an, trans. by Wu Ming, ISBN 0-936185-68-6

ACUTE ABDOMINAL SYN-DROMES: Their Diagnosis & Treatment by Combined Chinese-Western Medicine by Alon Marcus, ISBN 0-936185-31-7

AGING & BLOOD STASIS: A New Approach to TCM Geriatrics by Yan De-xin, ISBN 0-936185-63-5

AIDS & ITS TREATMENT ACCORDING TO TRADITIONAL CHINESE MEDICINE by Huang Bing-shan, trans. by Fu-Di & Bob Flaws, ISBN 0-936185-28-7

THE BOOK OF JOOK: Chinese Medicinal Porridges, An Alternative to the Typical Western Breakfast by B. Flaws, ISBN0-936185-60-0

CHINESE MEDICAL PALMIS-TRY: Your Health in Your Hand by Zong Xiao-fan & Gary Liscum, ISBN 0-936185-64-3

CHINESE MEDICINAL TEAS: Simple, Proven, Folk Formulas for Common Diseases & Promoting Health by Zong Xiao-fan & Gary Liscum, ISBN 0-936185-76-7

CHINESE MEDICINAL WINES & ELIXIRS by Bob Flaws, ISBN 0-936185-58-9

CHINESE PEDIATRIC MAS-SAGE THERAPY: *A Parent's & Practitioner's Guide to the Prevention & Treatment of Childhood Illness* by Fan Ya-li, ISBN 0-936185-54-6

CHINESE SELF-MASSAGE THE-RAPY: The Easy Way to Health by Fan Ya-li ISBN 0-936185-74-0

CLASSICAL MOXIBUSTION SKILLS in Clinical Practice by Sung Baek, ISBN 0-936185-16-3

A COMPENDIUM OF TCM PAT-TERNS & TREATMENTS by Bob Flaws & Daniel Finney, ISBN 0-936185-70-8

CURING ARTHRITIS NATURALLY WITH CHINESE MEDICINE by Doug Frank & Bob Flaws ISBN 0-936185-87-2

CURING PMS NATURALLY WITH CHINESE MEDICINE by Bob Flaws ISBN 0-936185-85-6

THE DAO OF INCREASING LONGEVITY AND CONSER-VING ONE'S LIFE by Anna Lin & Bob Flaws, ISBN 0-936185-24-4

THE DAO OF HEALTHY EATING ACCORDING TO CHINESE MEDICINE by Bob Flaws, ISBN 0-936185-92-9

THE DIVINELY RESPONDING CLASSIC: *A Translation of the Shen Ying Jing from Zhen Jiu Da Cheng*, trans. by Yang Shou-zhong & Liu Feng-ting ISBN 0-936185-55-4